Chimeras, Hybrids, and Interspecies Research

Chimeras, Hybrids, and Interspecies Research

Politics and Policymaking

Andrea L. Bonnicksen

Georgetown University Press • Washington, D.C.

Georgetown University Press, Washington, D.C.
www.press.georgetown.edu
© 2009 by Georgetown University Press. All rights
reserved.

Bonnicksen, Andrea L.
  Chimeras, hybrids, and interspecies research : politics
and policymaking / Andrea Bonnicksen.
       p. cm.
  Includes bibliographical references and index.
  ISBN 978-1-58901-574-6 (alk. paper)
  1. Mosaicism—Research—Government policy—
United States.   2. Transgenic animals—Research—
Government policy—United States.   I. Title.
  QH445.7.B66 2009
  174'.957—dc22
                                    2009007990

∞ This book is printed on acid-free paper meeting the
requirements of the American National Standard for
Permanence in Paper for Printed Library Materials.

15 14 13 12 11 10 09   9 8 7 6 5 4 3 2
First printing

Printed in the United States of America

To the Libbys
Linda, Russel, Michael, Russel Jr., Sheila, Jake, Morgan

Contents

Tables and Figures

Acknowledgments

I AM ESPECIALLY GRATEFUL TO Northern Illinois University for its program of Presidential Research Professorships. Receipt of one of these awards provided the budgetary support and released time that enabled me to write this book. Without the award, it would not have been written. I also extend grateful acknowledgment to John A. Robertson at the University of Texas at Austin, Bonnie Steinbock at SUNY Albany, and Robert H. Blank at the University of Canterbury for their help early in the research process.

I wish to thank Christopher M. Jones, chair of my department, for his support in accommodating my absence during a particularly busy year in the department. I owe special thanks to the Department of Bioethics and Humanities at the University of Washington and its chair, Wylie Burke, for arranging a Visiting Scholar affiliation during the 2006–2007 academic year. I also thank Michael A. Corn and Carol Ware at the University of Washington for their insightful comments. Mark S. Frankel at the American Association for the Advancement of Science and Jason Scott Robert at Arizona State University provided superb recommendations on reading earlier versions of the manuscript, and I am grateful for their direction. I thank Richard Brown, director of Georgetown University Press, for his encouragement; Nicole Kooistra, Jessica Jones, and Lauren Hall for their excellent research assistance; Neil Colwell for his original illustrations; and the tea ladies (Dorothy Coleman, Annette Johns, and Sharon Sytsma) for their good humor and support. For offering me wonderful house-sitting locations from which to write, I thank Linda Libby and Bobbi Malone.

Abbreviations

ART	assisted reproductive technology
ASRM	American Society for Reproductive Medicine
CIRM	California Institute for Regenerative Medicine
ES	embryonic stem [cell]
ESCRO	Embryonic Stem Cell Research Oversight [Committee]
ESHRE	European Society for Human Reproduction and Embryology
FDA	Food and Drug Administration
HERP	Human Embryo Research Panel
HFEA	Human Fertilisation and Embryology Authority
HFE Act	[U.K.] Human Fertilisation and Embryology [Act]
HNHI	human-nonhuman interspecific
HOP	hamster oocyte penetration [test]
IGM	inheritable genetic modification
iPS	induced pluripotent stem [cell]
ISSCR	International Society for Stem Cell Research
IRB	Institutional Review Board
ISR	interspecies research
IVF	in vitro fertilization
mtDNA	mitochondrial DNA
NBAC	National Bioethics Advisory Commission
NAS	National Academy of Sciences
PCB	President's Council on Bioethics
r-DNA	recombinant DNA
SCHB	Scottish Council on Human Bioethics
SCNT	somatic cell nuclear transfer

Introduction

AT ISSUE IN THIS BOOK are studies that combine genes, gametes, embryos, or embryonic stem (ES) cells from human and nonhuman species at the earliest stages of development. What is here called *early interspecies research* (ISR) involves the shared presence of human and/ or animal embryos and ES cells in a potentially inheritable way. The prospect of such studies has been flagged, whether justifiably or not, by a number of observers and policy makers as problematic.

One example of early ISR is the injection of human ES cells into a mouse blastocyst (four- to six-day embryo of approximately three hundred cells) in order to understand how human ES cells function over time in a living system. As the fetal mouse develops, the human cells differentiate and integrate. The ultimate goal is to understand the properties of ES cells better in order to develop cell-based therapies for humans. The recipient mice, studied before or after birth, would be chimeras, with some human cells existing side by side with mouse cells.

A second example is the substitution of animal eggs for human eggs in investigations geared to developing cell therapies for humans. In theory, if the nucleus from a patient's somatic cell is introduced to an enucleated egg, the egg can be stimulated to cleave and will yield an inner cell mass from which ES cells can be derived after about five days. These ES cells, which are capable of differentiating to virtually any type of body cell, can be coaxed to differentiate and used for cell replacement therapies. The goal is to derive ES cells that have the same genome as the patient who provided the nucleus. Many eggs would be needed in these preliminary studies, so investigators have proposed using animal eggs, which are abundant, in the early stages of research. The embryonic entity with a human nucleus and animal cytoplasm would be a cybrid or cytoplasmic hybrid.

Combining human and nonhuman cells is common in research, as when human cells are injected into adult mice to test a vaccine. *Early* ISR is used as a concept here to look beyond these traditional interspecies investigations in order to focus on studies that combine human and nonhuman embryos and/or ES cells in a way that could have a systemic effect on the organism if it were allowed to develop. Any studies using human embryos or ES cells have been contentious in the United States and other countries. The question here is whether pairing human and nonhuman biological material to produce such entities as chimeras or cybrids elevates the stakes by raising new and distinct ethical and policy issues. Exploring the dimensions of this research, regardless of the conclusions, helps to clarify recurring opposition to early ISR, as evidenced in preemptive restrictions in various countries and deliberations in the scholarly literature and in policy advisory groups.

From one point of view, the concept of early ISR is curious at best and unnecessarily provocative at worst. Whether the cell mix is all human, all animal, or a combination is, according to this view, insignificant. Of more importance is the purpose of studies and their feasibility, reliability, justification, and promise, all of which supersede distinctions about heritable human-nonhuman combinations. Here early ISR is not morally distinct, aside from underlying questions about whether human ES-cell research is appropriate in any form. If the human-nonhuman aspect is perceived as troublesome, efforts can be made to appease concerns. Lee Silver, a Princeton geneticist, typifies this perspective by positing that many scientists view early ISR as a red herring—much ado about very little. He predicts that members of society will take such interventions "in stride" and "continue to move along an orderly moral path" (Silver 2006, 187).

From a second point of view, the combined presence of nonhuman and human cells at the embryonic level is a clarion call for further attention. Here more than a difference of degree separates early ISR from ongoing research techniques. The mere combination is qualitatively different, and it poses implications for future and more problematic interchanges. Leon Kass, the first chair of George W. Bush's appointed President's Council on Bioethics, for example, points to a "growing number of experiments that are now putting human stem cells and their derivatives into animals to test them for . . . their therapeutic potential." He cautions that "it is not so much that science has raised new questions, but that it has made these old questions now urgent and very timely" (President's Council on Bioethics 2003b, 1–2).

To some extent, these perspectives reflect ideological differences about biotechnology in general. Disagreements about the promise or peril of biotechnology were felt and expressed in the early years of modern bio-technology following recombinant DNA discoveries in 1973 and the first birth of an infant from external fertilization in 1978. Observers pointed to genetic engineering, cloning, artificial wombs, and animal-human hybrids as potential applications that should give pause to the explo-ration of new technologies. These applications—called "aboriginal" by Eric Juengst for their conceptual presence at the beginning of modern biotechnology—helped to frame a specter of unacceptable reproductive outcomes down the road (Juengst 1991, 587). For example, when prepar-ing a report in the United States on reproductive technologies in 1979, the Ethics Advisory Board set up by the Department of Health, Education, and Welfare was warned of negative outcomes from in vitro fertiliza-tion, including the "formation of hybrids or chimeras (intraspecific and interspecific)" along with other deleterious outcomes (Ethics Advisory Board 1979, 173).

In the years since recombinant DNA research and in vitro fertiliza-tion commenced, much debate has surrounded two long-feared poten-tial applications of modern biotechnology: human germ line genetic modifications and cloning. Considerably less attention has been directed to animal-human hybrids, however. In the late 1970s and early 1980s, various nations, including Denmark, the United Kingdom, Germany, and Spain, initiated legal provisions forbidding various animal-human permutations. Denmark's 1987 law, for example, forbade experiments designed to enable "the production of living human beings who are hy-brids with a genetic constitution including components from other spe-cies" (Denmark 1988). The Parliamentary Assembly of the Council of Europe issued a Recommendation in 1986 on the use of human embryos and fetuses in research. In relevant part it called on member states to forbid implanting a human embryo into an animal uterus or vice versa, fusing human and animal gametes, or fusing embryos in such a way as to produce chimeras (Council of Europe 1986). These and other provisions were unusual because there was no clear need or urgency to limit such animal-human combinations.

Since the announced derivation of human ES cells in 1998, investigations into the properties and potential of human ES cells have brought some forms of human-nonhuman early ISR into the public debate. This recent interest in animal-human interventions in stem-cell research originally unfolded, in large part, in the academic context. Symposia in scholarly journals have provided a forum for academics to explore the ethical implications of early ISR (see, e.g., Robert and Baylis 2003; Austriaco 2006; Greely et al. 2007; Baylis and Robert 2007, 43; Baylis 2008). The growing list of other published articles makes the discourse more thorough and thoughtful than the brief discussions of thirty years ago. In addition policy advisory groups have weighed issues associated with early ISR and have made various recommendations about whether and how to manage concerns about the research. Two of the more visible reports are from the National Academy of Sciences (NAS) and the International Society for Stem Cell Research (ISSCR), both of which included provisions about early ISR in their recommendations about the ethical conduct of human ES-cell studies (Committee on Guidelines 2005; ISSCR 2006). In the United States, the California Institute for Regenerative Medicine and other agencies that fund human ES-cell research have also addressed early ISR in their funding guidelines (California Institute for Regenerative Medicine 2007).

In the more public venue, President George W. Bush surely startled many in his 2006 State of the Union speech by calling on the U.S. Congress to prohibit the "most egregious abuses of medical research" such as the "creation of animal-human hybrids" (State of the Union 2006). No front-page or headline event prompted this unusual passage, which was the president's sole reference to science in the speech and on which the president did not elaborate. The language echoed that of Eric Cohen, who wanted the administration to prevent the creation of human embryos for research and the degradation of human procreation that would come by "transgressing the species boundary between human and non-human life" (Cohen 2005, 3). It also evoked a 2004 report by the appointed President's Council on Bioethics (PCB), which recommended that Congress ban hybrid animal-human embryos to forestall actions by "some adventurous or renegade researchers" (President's Council on Bioethics 2004, 220).

Bernard Rollin calls it "bad ethical thinking" to "confus[e] whatever disturbs people with genuine ethical issues" (Rollin 2007b, 643). The fact that a possible practice offends some people, in other words, does not necessarily mean the practice raises substantial ethical issues. Rollin asserts that if scientists do not look much into the ethical implications of their research, this leaves a vacuum about ethical implications. The vacuum is soon "filled by doomsdayers, sectarian theologians, politicians, and others with claims that tend to be thrilling, lurid, and pretentious but are devoid of genuine ethical content" (644). When bad ethical thinking is in play, easy reliance on clichés and metaphors can override careful deliberations about the essence of issues.

Research involving early interspecies studies has its share of easy clichés that prompt one to question just how "genuine" the issues are. Certainly some concerns are sensational or even politically generated anxieties with little substantive content. But others, as evidenced by the deliberations of academics and policy advisory bodies in recent years, indicate a serious examination of expressed concerns. The goal of this book is to direct attention to germane policy questions and, in the process, to separate out issues that do not hold up as particularly useful or genuine. Its purpose is to add to the diverse voices in the public debate that reflect a different framing—one that aims for a more mundane rendering of the role of early ISR in contemporary research.

The recent reemergence of animal-human hybrids in public discourse points to the concept's resiliency. The cautions expressed about hybrids in 1979 were reiterated in 2008, when Adam Schulman wrote an introductory essay in a book on human dignity and bioethics commissioned by the PCB that referred to the "deliberate creation of animal-human chimeras" as the "most egregious abuses of the new biotechnologies" (Schulman 2008, 13). These cautions also appeared in antichimera bills introduced to Congress. One self-labeled biotechnology conservative advocated a "bioethics agenda" in the second term of the Bush administration that would place an emphasis on not crossing human-nonhuman species boundaries (Cohen 2005).

The generic animal-human hybrid concept evokes powerful imagery. For example, proposals to pair human cell nuclei and animal eggs were publicized in 1998 when the *Washington Post* reported that a biotechnology company had attempted to develop ES-cell lines by transferring the nucleus of a human cheek cell to an enucleated cow egg. The cleaving embryo (if it were in fact an embryo) would be destroyed after ES cells had been derived from the inner cell mass; it would not be transferred to a human for reproduction. Within thirty-six hours of the report, however, President Clinton contacted his newly created bioethics council, the National Bioethics Advisory Commission (NBAC), and asked it to consider the implications of this matter and to report to him "as soon as possible." Clinton wrote that he was "deeply troubled" by research "involving the mingling of human and non-human species." He saw this as the "creation of an embryonic stem cell that is part human and part cow" (Clinton 1998).

The staying power of the concept of animal-human hybrids suggests the symbolic resonance of interspecies studies, which appear to touch on values and interests regarded as worthy of protection. As noted by Murray Edelman, symbols fill a social need by drawing attention to developments that touch core values (Edelman 1995). The "framing" of issues may also be at work here, which is defined as the "process by which people develop a particular conceptualization of an issue" (Chong and Druckman 2007, 104). In public opinion polling it is well known that the framing of a question affects the response to it. In the political arena framing arises when those in or aspiring to public office try to "mobilize voters behind their policies by encouraging them to think about those policies along particular lines" (106). Repeated references to "animal-human hybrids" and "egregious research" in the early 2000s illustrate an attempt to frame the issue around, perhaps, mistrust of science. Framing has an impact. When studies about early ISR are targeted as problematic, this presents additional barriers for stem-cell investigations, which already face restrictive policies (Greely et al. 2007, 37).

This book differs from the literature on human-nonhuman chimeric research in two primary ways. First, most ethical and policy analyses to date focus on a single form of early ISR, usually chimeras. Yet laws, regulations, and proposed policies often group several types of early ISR under a common umbrella, such as provisions for both chimeras and hybrids in Canada's Assisted Human Reproduction Act (Canada/Government 2004). If these techniques are grouped together for policy purposes, it makes sense also to study them side by side in an examination of issues. In an effort to present an analysis with more nuances, the book divides ISR into five types, as described below. This presumes that not all early ISR is alike, and this presumption in turn paves the way for a comparison and contrast of the justifications and objections.

The book also differs from other analyses by examining objections in the public arena regardless of their implausibility; in other words, it considers realistic and sensational objections alike as long as one or more governments, not necessarily in the United States, have taken them seriously enough to have enacted regulations or prohibitions. It can be argued that taking sensational claims seriously is problematic because this act will in itself confer legitimacy on the claims (Greely et al. 2007, 28). It is counterargued, however, that because policies have already been proposed and developed on the basis of at times sensational scenarios, the weakly grounded objections have already been accorded some degree of legitimacy. Ignoring them leaves ill-formed opinions unchallenged, whereas a closer look at the techniques and concerns, which this book aims to take, confronts those perceptions.

WHAT IS EARLY ISR?

As stated above, "general" ISR, which is not as a rule morally problematic, encompasses research and therapies that combine human-nonhuman DNA, cells, tissues, or organs without involving human embryos or potentially inheritable modifications. Examples are using pig valves to treat humans whose heart valves no longer function or mice with human skin or muscle. These studies generate few issues outside those raised for xenotransplantation generally. "Early" ISR, in contrast, involves human-nonhuman cell transfer at the earliest, prenatal, stages of development. It involves gametes, embryos, or human ES cells, and it can lead to inheritable modifications.

Inquiry into early ISR is complicated by the interchangeable use of terms such as hybrids and chimeras, which in fact refer to different scientific techniques. A bill introduced to the U.S. Congress, for example, listed eight meanings of chimeras, including what were technically hybrids (U.S. Senate 2005b). When President George W. Bush referred to animal-human hybrids in his speech, he probably meant stem-cell chimeras, but this was not clear in his comments (Elias 2006; Moreno 2006). Definitions challenged a committee in the U.K. House of Commons as it sought to understand what the government meant by "hybrid and chimera embryos" (U.K. House of Commons 2007, 44). Sometimes definitions are lacking altogether or are vague. For example, the pharmaceutical company Geron set up an Ethics Advisory Board that published a report specifying voluntary restrictions for human ES-cell research. In relevant part, it stated that the research "will not involve any cloning for purposes of human reproduction, any transfer to a uterus, or any creation of chimeras," but it did not clarify what it meant by creating chimeras (Geron Ethics Advisory Board 1999, 31).

Ambiguity arises in artistic endeavors as well. A key orienting image is that of the mythological Greek chimera, an ill-tempered creature made up of part goat, serpent, and lion. This chimera mixes three animal species, whereas other chimeras—"centaurs, sphinxes, werewolves, minotaurs and mermaids, and the gorgon Medusa"—are all part human and thus more apropos for recent concerns (Wade 2005, D1). Moreover, this ancient mythological symbol pales beside renderings in contemporary culture of interspecies chimeras, hybrids, and transgenics that pique the contemporary imagination and speak to some of the same uncertainties as the Greek chimera. In her exhibit, "We Are Family," the artist Patricia Piccinini features a life-size sculpture of a hairless part human and part dog mother suckling her pups/babies. The posture, litter, and floppy ears are reminiscent of a dog but the faces, body parts, and pale skin are human-like (Piccinini 2003). The vision is unsettling. It is unclear what techniques are symbolically depicted in Piccinini's work. Are the mother and offspring animal-human hybrids created by pairing human and canine gametes? Or are they transgenic dogs with human DNA liberally spliced in? Or could they be chimeras, created from the fusion of human and canine embryos and with cells from both species filtering like a mosaic throughout the bodies? Piccinini is not accountable for answers; she is, after all, an artist with intentions other than scientific precision. Yet the sculptures cause one to wonder how these creatures would have been created if they were living beings rather than works of silicone and fiberglass. The underlying method—albeit imaginary—is confusing, as it is surely meant to be.

Contemporary images at once invite curiosity and discussion, which is a welcome effect, and risk distorting the science involved, which is a less welcome effect. Art plays a key role in public discourse in that a painting of an animal-human chimera can "facilitate discussion of the issue long before such a creature has been created in reality" (Andrews n.d.). Visual images are "more accessible than scientific publications," and they "turn the technical talk of science into the emotional domain of public discourse" (Anker and Nelkin 2004, 4). As Edelman puts it, art gives "cognitive and emotional resonances" to political actions (Edelman 1995, 6). Although artistic rendering plays a part in public deliberations, it is a dubious basis for policy making. It is one thing to visit a museum and come out musing, "What *were* those things?" It is another to impute reality to the sculptures and call for regulations as a result. Reflecting and giving voice to concerns are different endeavors than shaping policy responses to those concerns.

Both scientific and social definitions apply to early ISR (Board on Life Sciences and Board on Health Sciences Policy 2004, 6). A scientific definition of a chimera can be this: an organism with cells from two genetically different sets of parents in its body. A social definition can be this: an animal with cut and pasted body parts reminiscent of the Greek chimera. According to Rollin, although the social definition may be technically incorrect, when it is buoyed by values and emotion, it may turn out to be the more "significant for an ethical or moral analysis" (Board on Life Sciences and Board on Health Sciences Policy 2004, 6).

As indicated above, this book distinguishes among five types of ISR. Each type meets two criteria. First, each is characterized as early ISR, involving human-nonhuman cell or DNA transfer at the earliest stages of development. Second, each has been on the policy agenda at one time or another. This means it has been a problem to which people inside or outside the government have paid "some serious attention at any given time" and have devoted time and effort to influencing the policy process (Kingdon 1984, 3). Attempted influence includes proposals such as U.S. Senate Bill 659, the Human Chimera Prohibition Act of 2005 (U.S. Senate 2005a). Completed influence includes actual policy decisions such as the United Kingdom's Human Fertilisation and Embryology Act (HFE Act) 2008 (U.K. HFE Act 2008). Policy is broadly defined to include both governmental and nongovernmental decisions that serve as a guide to action. Policy derived from statutes, administrative codes, and recommendations by government-sponsored advisory bodies is public policy. Policy developed in the private sector, which includes clinical practices, recommendations by privately sponsored advisory bodies, and guidance documents from professional associations, is private policy (Bonnicksen 2002, 4).

Methods that come within the umbrella of early ISR are presumed to be distinct and worthy of separate analysis for the ethical and policy issues they raise. Looking at techniques individually has the merit of encouraging precision and guarding against clichés and overgeneralizations. On the other hand, it is important not to pay so much attention to distinctions of technique that larger issues are lost. Moreover, distinctions can distort how cell biology is viewed, making it seem more capable of being "scientifically parsed" than it really is (Association of American Medical Colleges 2005, 31).

The typology of early ISR identified for this book is briefly presented here:

- *Chimeras* are created by combining cells from two genetically different individuals. This can be done in various ways, including the injection of human ES cells into nonhuman blastocysts. Chimeras are created at various stages of development. For example, human ES cells or their derivatives can be transferred to nonhuman embryos, fetuses, neonates, or adults.
- *Animal-human hybrids* would theoretically be created by fertilizing a human egg with a nonhuman spermatozoan or a nonhuman egg with a human spermatozoan. It is highly unlikely a hybrid embryo could be gestated to birth; nevertheless, hybrids invoke vivid imagery in the public imagination and appear in policy proposals. They can range from a real but unproblematic

manipulation (the human-hamster fertility assay or "hamster test") to the fanciful "humanzee," a creature eyed metaphorically as the worst kind of hybrid.

- *Cybrids* are created by transferring a human cell nucleus to an enucleated animal egg in order to derive ES cells and to study other features of developmental biology. Also called cytoplasmic hybrid embryos in public debate, they are called here cybrids, following informal use of this term in the United Kingdom.

- *Cross-species embryo transfer* refers to the transfer of a human embryo to a nonhuman uterus or the transfer of a nonhuman embryo to a human uterus. Although unlikely, such transfers have been the subject of national laws and policy proposals.

- *Nonhuman-human transgenics* refers to splicing human DNA to nonhuman embryos, which is common, or nonhuman DNA to human embryos, which is not on the horizon.

The selection of these particular techniques reflects current topics raised in the ethics and policy literature. Each may be assumed to be transitory; given rapid scientific and technological changes, a chimeric technique today may be outdated tomorrow. As much as possible, then, it is useful to identify issues that will likely reappear even as individual techniques change. The labels are faulty in the way they evoke the equivalent of three apples (chimeras, hybrids, cybrids) with two oranges (cross-species embryo transfer and transgenics), with the first three referring to entities and the second two to processes. This is akin to referring to "test tube babies" as entities and "in vitro fertilization" as a process. The first is a short-hand reference to the outcome, whereas the second is a reference to the process. In the following chapters all five techniques are meant to refer to processes aimed at scientific ends. "Chimeras," "hybrids," and "cybrids" are part of the research process geared to understanding various facets of biological development.

WHAT ETHICAL OBJECTIONS ARE RAISED AGAINST EARLY ISR?

Numerous objections have been raised in regard to early ISR (see, e.g., Baylis and Robert 2007, 205). The debate has been vigorous at times;

for example, one set of observers noted how much more discussion was generated in the United States than had been expected over proposals to transfer human ES-cell-derived neurons to mouse brains (Greely et al. 2007, 37). To provide a structure to the inquiry here, three commonly expressed objections are examined: (1) early ISR is an affront to human dignity (perhaps the most frequently invoked objection), (2) unwelcome births will follow such as the birth of beings that combine observable human and nonhuman features, and (3) early ISR will blur distinctions between species and lead to moral confusion as a result. Each is briefly described here.

Thinking about Dignity

The concept of dignity is frequently invoked in discussions about early ISR. For example, Josephine Johnston and Christopher Eliot regard affronts to human dignity as a meaningful objection to the creation of human-nonhuman chimeras, and they urge further examination of the ways dignity might be violated by the creation of beings with part human and part animal characteristics (Johnston and Eliot 2003; see also Baylis and Fenton 2007). Adam Schulman regards dignity as "establish[ing] a baseline of inviolable rights—in effect, a floor of decency beneath which no treatment of human beings should ever sink" (Schulman 2008, 13). He points to the "deliberate creation of animal-human chimeras" as a practice that would fall below this floor (13). He asks, "Would it not be degrading to our humanity and an affront to human dignity to produce animal-human chimeras with some human features and some features of lower animals?" (17). In Schulman's meaning dignity relates to the "essential and inviolable core of our *humanity*" (17) and the human attributes that are "considered inviolable." Human dignity can but must not be abridged by biotechnology, according to this perspective. These authors frame the concept in a way that makes it appear they have in mind fully developed beings rather than microscopic entities, but in discussions that refer to chimeras or hybrids generally, this distinction is not always clear. The point is that the authors are concerned about the impact on human dignity, whether from the creation of embryos or by the thought of fully developed beings.

Dignity also justified U.S. Senate Bill 659, which would have banned human-human and animal-human chimeras because they would threaten "respect for human dignity and the integrity of the human species" (U.S. Senate 2005a). A bill introduced to the Delaware legislature that would ban cloning between humans and nonhumans stated that techniques to "create human/non-human embryos . . . represent a fundamental threat to human dignity and integrity" (Delaware General Assembly 2007). Here it is clear the bill's authors had in mind embryos as well as fully developed organisms. In the United Kingdom, the Scottish Council of Human Bioethics asserted that "the creation of certain kinds of human-nonhuman embryonic combinations could seriously undermine the whole concept of human dignity" (quoted in U.K. House of Commons 2007, 24). The Science and Technology Committee of the U.K. House of Commons observed that the human dignity argument "formed the basis for much of the opposition evidence we have received" in response to its inquiry about the use of cybrids (U.K. House of Commons 2007, 24).

Dignity can be defined in many ways. Cynthia Cohen, for example, refers to a "family or cluster of capacities" associated with being human, such as communication at a sophisticated level, ability to display empathy, and involvement in social relations (Cohen 2007b, 125). Some humans have many of these capacities, and others have fewer, but all enjoy an association with being human. Martha Nussbaum recognizes the inviolable worth of humans, based on their capabilities, which include trained and untrained capacities (Nussbaum 2008). Human dignity "requires creating the conditions in which capacities can develop and unfold themselves."

Human dignity has a long tradition in bioethics, dating in particular to the "intrinsic worth of all humans" embraced in the 1948 Universal Declaration on Human Rights, which "acknowledges the 'inherent dignity' and 'equal and inalienable rights of all members of the human family'" (Caulfield and Brownsword 2006, 72). It is held to be "one of the most common concerns raised in public debates, academic arguments . . . and policy documents" about biotechnology (Johnston and Eliot 2003). The Second World Conference on Bioethics in 2002 reiterated the "universal commitment" to dignity as an "attribute of humankind" (Johnston and Eliot 2003). This highlights dignity as a precept of humanity in general.

Many defend the concept of dignity as useful for evaluating the morality of biotechnologies, whereas others criticize its use as an evaluative concept, saying it is vague and can conveniently take on whatever meaning the person using it wants it to take (Macklin 2003; President's Council on Bioethics 2005b, 2; Pinker 2008, 30). Caulfield and Brownsword claim its meaning has taken on political overtones as it is used as a "dubious justification for policies that are aimed at constraining controversial biotechnologies" (Caulfield and Brownsword 2006, 72). Ruth Macklin regards dignity as a superfluous concept when autonomy, which requires that no one may arbitrarily intrude on one's body or freedom, is the core of what is to be protected for humans (Macklin 2003). Here dignity is an "engine of individual empowerment, reinforcing individual autonomy and the right to self-determination" (Caulfield and Brownsword 2006, 72). This highlights dignity as it applies like autonomy to individual humans in a medical setting.

It is not the intention in this book to enter the spirited debate about the use of dignity or to use a single definition in the following chapters. Still, in view of challenges to early ISR on dignity grounds, it is necessary to address these claims. In some cases the link between early ISR and human dignity is explicitly stated, as in assertions that creating a primate with significant human cognitive capacity through the transfer of human ES cells to the primate's fetal brain would violate human dignity because it would create a being with human-like attributes and deny that being the opportunity (if caged, for example) to exercise these attributes (Working Group on Interspecific Chimeric Brains 2005; Streiffer 2005). In other cases the link is left unclear beyond a general assertion that the creation of chimeras or hybrids would violate human dignity.

Because the claims are not always explicit, the discussion in the following chapters takes an exploratory posture and asks for each technique what *could* be meant by an intrusion on dignity. This will necessarily be speculative, but it is meant to acknowledge the argument and fill in gaps. If the claim is not persuasive, this reflects weaknesses in the merit of using human dignity to evaluate the ethical dimensions of early ISR (see also Melo-Martin 2008).

Thinking about Procreation

One concern about early ISR is that basic research today on embryos will lead to unsavory "next steps" related to procreation tomorrow. The stage is set, the argument goes, for the creation of entities with traits reminiscent of humans, including appearance, cognition, and behavior. This concern has been expressed about animals at different places on the evolutionary ladder, ranging from a "humanized mouse" (mouse with human neural attributes) to a humanzee (cross breeding of a human and chimpanzee). The vision of "creating some sort of creature that would be functioning like a human being and yet having very strong animal-like behaviors" (Lamb 2005, 1) is not surprising given that whole beings such as chimeras, centaurs, and gorgons are represented in art, mythology, and literature. Even though we know intellectually that such beings will not come to be, they supply "images that construct the worlds in which we act" (Edelman 1995, 3).

Concerns for a nonhuman being with human traits and for a human being with nonhuman traits have been raised in the policy arena. In a meeting of the PCB to discuss chimeras in research, Kass started the session by asking why it would be wrong to create a humanzee (President's Council on Bioethics 2003b, 2). He did not necessarily believe that a humanzee would ever be created, but he wanted to examine the most extreme scenario first in order to refine arguments for more realistic prospects. Johnstone and Eliot note that "intentionally creating human beings or part-human beings that possess compromised humanness" is an objection in research using chimeras (Johnston and Eliot 2003, 2).

Thinking about Species

A third expressed concern is that human-nonhuman studies will challenge traditional notions about species boundaries in a way that treads on human interests (Robert and Baylis 2003; Karpowicz, Cohen, and van der Kooy 2005). Jason Robert and Francoise Baylis, for example, argue that chimeric research may cause moral confusion if it dilutes the boundaries that humans believe separate species and help order the world. The authors are not necessarily troubled by moral confusion per se, but they believe that it, of all the arguments raised against the creation of human-nonhuman chimeras, is "the most plausible objection" (Robert and Baylis 2003, 44).

Although most critical commentaries on early ISR relate to the impact of the studies on the human species, some observers look to potentially deleterious impacts on animal well-being. Whereas in most cases impact on animal well-being is likely to be minimal (for example, destroying mouse embryos, fetuses, and neonates before appreciable consciousness develops), concern has also been leveled at more significant effects. For example, a multidisciplinary group that weighed the moral issues of grafting human ES cells or neural progenitor cells to developing nonhuman primates asked whether grafting would "make the brain more human-like" and affect "animal cognition, emotion, or behavior" (Working Group on Interspecific Chimeric Brains 2005; see also Greene et al. 2005). Harm to the animals would be more pronounced if the living conditions of the animals were not modified to reflect their enhanced cognition (Working Group on Interspecific Chimeric Brains 2005; Streiffer 2005).

Thinking about the nonhuman species in early ISR brings to mind a compelling series of bat photographs in a book by Lorraine Daston and Gregg Mitman (2005). When bats are viewed in their usual position, hanging upside down on a branch, they suggest to us weirdness, the darkness of caves, and flitting motions. But when viewed in photographs rotated 180° to display them so that they appear to be standing upright on a branch, bats wrong side up reveal themselves as different animals altogether—delicate creatures with round eyes and wings demurely pulled across their chins, much like a line of lithe ballet dancers waiting to go on-stage. The authors wanted to encourage thinking *with* rather than *about* animals, and the upended photos help the viewer to see these animals in a totally different perspective. Analogously, exploring the impact of early ISR may encourage a more careful look at the interests of both parties in interspecies studies.

WHAT ISSUES WARRANT ELEVATION
TO THE POLICY AGENDA?

Policy development is based on a long process of "softening up" in which "ideas are floated, bills introduced, speeches made; proposals are drafted, then amended in response to reaction and floated again" (Kingdon 1984, 123). John Kingdon writes, "the more a proposal is discussed, the more seriously it is taken" (148). When a matter such as early ISR arises, debate, deliberation, and education are all part of a robust discussion. This means that conceivably a range of matters will be taken seriously and will be on the policy agenda. Yet some of these matters will be more "agenda-worthy" than others. Generally these more compelling matters will have one or more focusing events that bring imminence to the issue. For example in the United Kingdom in 2006, researchers presented two protocols to the U.K. Human Fertilisation and Embryology Authority that would involve creating cybrids. This focusing event set in motion deliberations about a particular policy problem—whether cybrids are embryos under the HFE Act of 1990—and led to the eventual revision of relevant portions of that Act in 2008. In the United States Pierre Soupart at Vanderbilt University submitted a research protocol in 1977 involving in vitro fertilization (IVF), which set in motion the establishment of the Ethics Advisory Board, mandated by law to convene to weigh ethical issues before IVF research could be funded.

A matter is a contender for the policy agenda if it represents a problem and not just a condition. According to Kingdon, conditions turn into problems "when we come to believe that we should do something about them" (Kingdon 1984, 115). This is more likely when conflicting values are at issue and also when a focusing event occurs. Defining something as a problem matters: those benefiting from the status quo will shy away from identifying new problems; whereas those favoring policy change will attempt to identify problems in order to mobilize remedial action (115).

Other conditions that help elevate a matter to the policy agenda include the presence of a policy community of people willing to "invest their resources—time, energy, reputation, and sometimes money—in the hope of a future return." They also include the presence of policy alternatives and a receptive national mood (defined as a "rather large number of people out in the country . . . thinking along certain common lines") (Kingdon 1984, 129, 153). The likelihood of a matter being on the policy agenda is, in short, greater when a perceived problem, receptive national mood, and community of visible participants converge at once (206–9).

This book questions the extent to which early ISR raises problems that warrant significant remedial policy action. The U.S. oversight system for human ES-cell research heretofore has been minimal, in part because the federal government's involvement with the funding of human ES-cell research has been minimal. Nevertheless, the rudiments of a decentralized and largely voluntary policy have emerged from several sources since the

1998 announcement that human ES cells had been derived and cultured. In addition to regulations in place for research in general, ES-cell policies are based on (1) National Institutes of Health (NIH) guidelines, (2) state policies relating to research on human embryos, (3) recommendations by the Committee on Guidelines of the National Academy of Sciences, (4) guidelines developed by Embryonic Stem Cell Research Oversight (ESCRO) committees, and (5) long-standing norms respected by professional associations and policy advisory groups relating to human embryo research. All of these are foundations for developing norms and practices for early ISR as well.

Regarding the policy contribution of the NIH, early guidelines were minimal by virtue of President Bush's Executive Order in 2001 limiting funding to a small number of ES-cell lines that had been derived before August 9, 2001 (National Institutes of Health. Office of the Director 2001). This policy stipulated that the embryos must have been donated by couples who no longer needed them for their fertility efforts, had given informed consent to donate, and had not been offered "financial inducements" to donate.

One of President Barack Obama's first actions after taking office in 2009 was to lift the requirement that only cell lines derived by the 2001 date could be funded (White House 2009). Obama also directed the NIH to produce guidelines for human ES-cell research by mid-2009. Draft guidelines, made available for public comment in April 2009 and finalized after public comment to be effective on July 7, 2009, added new stipulations, particularly those related to informed consent (National Institutes of Health 2009). In addition, they included two provisions about early ISR that would make studies ineligible for funding: (1) no human ES cells or induced pluripotent stem cells (iPS) were to be introduced to nonhuman primate blastocysts, and (2) animals were not to be bred if the addition of human ES or iPS cells "may contribute to the germ line" (National Institutes of Health 2009).

The states provide a second source of U.S. policy. By 2007 in the United States, ten states had set up stem-cell programs or regenerative medicine institutes to encourage and/or fund ES-cell research (Hanna 2007; Vestal 2007). For example New Jersey set aside $10 million in 2004 for stem-cell research to be allocated over a period of ten years, and it allocated more funds later to construct a facility for the studies (Vestal 2007, 2). A successful ballot proposition in California in 2004 provided for $3 billion to be available over a ten-year period for stem-cell investigations. Aside from California, however, accompanying oversight policies in the states have not included specific provisions for early ISR (Lomax and Stayn 2008). It should also be noted that although some states have encouraged research using human ES cells, others have passed or attempted to pass laws restricting human embryo research in general or particular forms such as SCNT research (Okie 2005; Lomax and Stayn 2008; Dewan 2009). In these states, early ISR is unlikely to pass muster.

A third component of U.S. policy is a set of recommendations from a report in 2005 written by the Committee on Guidelines for Human Embryonic Stem Cell Research (hereafter Committee on Guidelines), written under the auspices of the National Research Council and Institute of Medicine. These facilities are two branches of the National Academy of Science, a nongovernmental organization charted by Congress to provide scientific advice to the Congress. In relevant part, the Committee on Guidelines recommended that institutions engaged in human ES-cell research set up ESCROs to add a layer of review beyond that provided by Institutional Review Boards (IRBs) in light of the "complex issues raised by hES cell research" (Committee on Guidelines 2005, 4). The report also included provisions relating to early ISR, as summarized in Table i.1 and discussed later.

Although the NAS is not a governmental agency, nor does it have enforcement power, the 2005 guidelines are regarded as "binding" by "many States, members of the press and many academic journals" (Association of American Medical Colleges 2005, 24). The guidelines have "offered a common set of ethical standards for a field that, due to the absence of comprehensive federal funding, was lacking national standards for research." These guidelines are periodically revisited and amended (National Research Council 2007; National Research Council 2008). The report from the Committee on Guidelines was preceded and influenced by guidelines established in the United Kingdom, Canada, and Australia (Hanna 2007, 130). In turn the report has provided a model for the development of "nearly identical" ES-cell policy recommendations in California and for the nongovernmental ISSCR (130).

Table i.1.   **Recommendations Relating to Early ISR in NAS Report**

Should be permitted only after review and approval by an ESCRO	Should not be permitted at this time
Introducing human ES cells into "non-human animals at any stage of embryonic, fetal, or postnatal development"	Introducing human ES cells into nonhuman primate blastocysts
	Introducing animal or human ES cells into human blastocysts
	Breeding animals into which human ES cells have been introduced at any stage
Areas of particular attention	Human nuclei and nonhuman eggs
Attention should be given to the "probable pattern and effects of differentiation and integration of the human cells into the nonhuman animal tissues"	Combining human nuclei and nonhuman eggs [cybrids] is a "potentially valuable research tool," but further investigation is needed about feasibility
Attention is needed if "human neuronal cells might participate in 'higher-order' brain functions in a nonhuman animal"	These entities should not be kept cleaving beyond fourteen days
Informed consent	Preparatory research
The informed consent process for donating embryos should include a statement that human ES cells from the embryos might be used for research in which the cells are genetically altered or in which human and nonhuman cells are mixed in animal models	Transfer of human ES cells to blastocysts from large mammals needs to be clearly justified
	Research involving transfer of nonhuman primate ES cells to mouse blastocysts should precede transfer of human ES cells to mouse blastocysts (34)

Source: Committee on Guidelines 2005, 33–35, 107–8, 111.

A fourth element of U.S. policy is the expanding network of ESCROs, which consider whether and how to monitor various research activities (O'Rourke, Abelman, and Herrernan 2007). Individual ESCROs, in touch via regional meetings, and other mechanisms, play a role in the development of guidelines for variations in human ES-cell research. Some ESCROs refer to early ISR (421). The stem-cell research oversight committee at the University of Wisconsin, for example, in 2008 covered human ES-cell research and also the "introduction of human pluripotent stem cells, or their derivatives, obtained from a non-embryonic source, into non-human animals at any embryonic, fetal, or postnatal stage, if an expected effect is that human cells will be integrated into the central nervous system, testes, or ovaries of the animal" (University of Wisconsin Stem Cell and Regenerative Medicine Center 2008).

A fifth component of U.S. policy is a set of norms about research involving human embryos generally respected by professionals, policy advisory groups, and investigators in the United States and other countries. These norms reflect the assumption that the human embryo is a "potential human being worthy of special respect" (Ethics Advisory Board 1979; Ethics Committee of the American Fertility Society 1986). Among other things, the embryo is regarded as having a "special status but not the same status as a living child or adult" (U.K. Department of Health 2000a, sec. 4.6). It is a "special biological entity" with a "specific symbolic significance," and society has an interest in protecting it (ESHRE Task Force 2001, 1046–7). It is entitled to "respect beyond that accorded to an embryo of other species" (U.K. Department of Health 2000a, sec. 4.6).

Sample norms, summarized in table i.2, reflect guidelines published by nongovernmental associations such as the American Society for Reproductive Medicine (ASRM), the European Society for Human Reproduction and Embryology (ESHRE), and the NAS. The principles appear, with variations, in public laws in the United Kingdom, Canada, Australia, and other countries, and they reiterate reports on embryo research dating to the 1980s (Walters 1987). A report of stem-cell policies in fifty countries indicates that eight forbid all human ES-cell research, seven permit the creation of embryos for research with provisions, and the others allow donated embryos with provisions (International Stem Cell Forum 2006, 366). The countries that allow research do so with "shared principles as well as professional norms and substantive and procedural conditions that further [beyond regulations] constrain this work" (366).

Conferences, symposia, scientific publications, institutional review boards, and professional associations all currently provide forums for policymaking when new issues arise regarding research on human embryos (Committee on Guidelines 2005, 12). As Hanna describes it, the 5,500 IRBs in the United States, together with professional societies, tangential laws, and "numerous publications," form the basis for regulating ES-cell research (Hanna 2007, 135). This leaves room to incorporate practices in response to new technologies and discoveries.

It is important to note that this book assumes in principle the ethical acceptability of using human embryos in research provided norms of research such as those in table i.2 are respected. To assume this baseline of acceptable research is to shift from debates over the ethics of embryo research, which have been abundantly covered in the literature, to questions about the ethics of early ISR in particular. Are these studies qualitatively different from studies using only human embryos and ES cells? How significant is the nonhuman component? Does the animal presence necessitate new practices and/or regulations?

The following chapters identify objections raised about early ISR in an effort to determine where policy attention is needed. Each chapter reviews the issues and asks how imminent the technique is and whether evidence exists of harm and/or benefit. In 1994 for example the Human Embryo Research Panel (HERP), set up by the NIH, categorized dimensions of research involving human embryos as ethically acceptable for federal funding, meriting "special consideration," or not ethically acceptable (National Institutes of Health 1994). One of the ten unacceptable techniques was the creation of a human-human chimera. Panel member Ronald Green later noted that within the unacceptable category, the human-human chimera was the "one to which we gave the least thought" (Green 2001, 100). This was not surprising given the absence of proposals or even academic deliberations about human chimeras, which signaled it was not a policy problem. The HERP's charge was to identify forms of embryo research that were ethically acceptable, and the members did not devote time to a vague and distant possibility. They did, however, give human-human chimeras a place on a policy grid that could be revisited later.

Chapter 1 covers the technique that has generated substantial ethical commentary—the use of human-nonhuman chimeras in basic research. Chapter 2 examines animal-human hybrids, which are at once the most fanciful of the five but also the concept that has generated the most colorful images and powerful metaphors. Because animal-human hybrids are not on the horizon, this chapter is necessarily short. Chapter 3 combines three techniques that have arisen in policy circles but that have not captured the public imagination to the same degree as have chimeras and hybrids. These are cybrids, cross-species embryo transfer, and transgenics. For organizational purposes these three techniques are grouped into a single chapter.

Table i.2. **Selected Norms for Research Using Human Embryos**

Selected norms and rules	Sample source of recommended rules
Prior studies on animals or human gametes should be conducted prior to using human embryos	National Institutes of Health 1994 ESHRE Task Force 2001
Embryos should be used only if there is "no satisfactory alternative" or if "no alternative more acceptable methods are available"	Ethics Committee of the ASRM 1997
The smallest possible number of embryos should be used	National Institutes of Health 1994 Ethics Committee of the ASRM 1997
The "investigator bears the burden of justifying the worthiness of the research"	Ethics Committee of the ASRM 1997 Committee on Guidelines 2005 ISSCR 2006
Research must be "scientifically valid and likely to produce scientific or clinical benefit"; "important clinical data" are expected to accrue	National Institutes of Health 1994 Ethics Committee of the ASRM 1997
Research must be conducted by qualified personnel in an "appropriate research setting"	National Institutes of Health 1994
Research proposals must be reviewed by an IRB or equivalent body	National Institutes of Health 1994 Ethics Committee of the ASRM 1997
Donated embryos should be used only with informed consent, including awareness of the nature of the studies	Ethics Committee of the ASRM 1997 Committee on Guidelines 2005 ISSCR 2006
Embryos should be created for research only if the information cannot be obtained from embryos donated by couples in fertility clinics	ESHRE Task Force 2001
Embryos must not be kept in vivo for more than fourteen days or beyond the beginning of the primitive streak, "whichever comes first"	National Institutes of Health 1994 Ethics Committee of the ASRM 1997 Committee on Guidelines 2005
Embryos must not be bought or sold	Ethics Committee of the ASRM 1997
Embryos used for research should not be transferred for pregnancy	ESHRE 2001

For each of the five types of early ISR, a rationale is given in the following chapters for pursuing the research. This can take a stretch of the imagination; for example, it is maddening to try to imagine a realistic rationale for transferring a nonhuman embryo to a woman's uterus. Nevertheless, nations have in fact barred transferring an animal embryo to a woman's uterus, so this has been a policy issue at one time or another. In each chapter ethical issues are discussed, illustrative policies are highlighted, and the "problem" status is assessed for the techniques involved.

Chapter 4 asks what motivates objections to combining human and animal biological material in basic research. Assuming that fundamental ideological differences are at play, it suggests that views about early ISR reflect different values related to orientation to biotechnology, wisdom about intuitive reactions, ability to draw lines, and differences between human and nonhuman species.

The conclusion looks at similarities and differences among the types of early ISR. It pursues the theme that research labeled animal-human is too easily ostracized without substantial reasons. Early ISR is met with often inchoate concerns rather than substantial risks or demonstrable harms, and it is questionable whether early ISR brings the urgency and advocacy requisite for significant policy change. This does not negate the importance of working to clarify techniques and goals and to provide forums for examining objections (Committee on Guidelines 2005, 41). It does, however, encourage deliberation so that policy development will be based on clearly articulated reasons and pragmatic queries with sufficient scientific input. In the process the impact of early ISR on human interests will be examined, along with the impact on ways of thinking about human and animal interests in tandem.

When the PCB was weighing chimeras at a meeting called for that purpose, conversation lapsed into discussions of humanzees, and Michael Gazzaniga commented that this subject was for people who have too much time on their hands (President's Council on Bioethics 2003b, 7, 9). He preferred an approach based on a "very limited, sober, biomedical question" rather than something sensational and of science fiction quality. Interspecies beings potentially include chimeras, animal-human hybrids, HNHIs (human-nonhuman interspecifics), and mosaics, and they provoke an unusually imaginative literature and artistic corpus from antiquity that has spanned millennia. Add to this H. G. Wells' beast people, Eduardo Kac's fluorescent green rabbit, Dean Koontz's primate/human Outsider, and, more recently, Michael Crichton's humanzee, and it is small wonder that confusion flows (Koontz 1987; Wells 1993; Kac [2000?]; Crichton 2006). Images in popular culture succeed in attracting attention; HNHIs fade in competition with humanzees, chimphumans, geeps, tigons, and zonkeys. With the serious business of biomedical research and useful policy at root, however, efforts to explore the techniques of research and to identify and engage arguments concerning its parameters may be welcome.

Chimeras

THE IMAGE OF THE MYTHOLOGICAL chimera, a "symbolic monster composed of incongruous parts," orients our minds to the idea of mixed parts coddled together (Anker and Nelkin 2004, 82). Although chimeras in ancient Greece were regarded as "dangerous, formidable, and powerful beasts, representing fantastic yet uncivilized and chaotic forces in nature that confronted mankind," chimeras in art today present more benign personas. Thomas Grunfeld's *Misfit (St. Bernard)*, a painting of a placid St. Bernard with a sheep's head, is regarded as a "classic chimera" (Anker and Nelkin 2004, 81, 108). Similarly, Stephan Balkenhol's *Three Hybrids, 1995* features three wood animal/men with the heads of a cow, a mouse, and a hawk and the bodies of humans (Balkenhol 1995). Even though the artist calls them hybrids, his creatures resemble the image of chimeras as cut and pasted beings. Far from monstrous, they wear corduroy trousers and project amiable dispositions.

Just as chimeras have different meanings in the world of art, so too do they convey different meanings in the world of science, with molecular biologists, geneticists, cell biologists, embryologists, and other academic specialists attaching somewhat different definitions (Karpowicz, Cohen, and van der Kooy 2005, 109–10; U.K. House of Commons 2007, 45). Broadly speaking a chimera is an organism with cells from "different embryonic origins" (Streiffer 2005, 347) or, similarly, "an organism composed of cells derived from at least two genetically different zygotes," which could be from the same or different species (National Institutes of Health 1994, 102).

There is no archetypal chimera, and chimeras take many forms, depending on the type of biological matter transferred (somatic cells, reproductive cells, individual ES cells, the entire inner cell mass of an embryo) and the stage of development of the recipient organism (pre-embryo, embryo after gastrulation, fetus, neonate, adult animal) (Greely 2003). Some chimeras are intraspecies, and others are interspecies. Some are born naturally, and others are created through human intervention (see figure 1.1 on p. 39).

"Trace" chimeras result when only a limited number of human cells are introduced, and they are introduced after the stage when cells would affect the germ line (DeGrazia 2007, 309). Here the integration of cells is minimal (ISSCR 2006, 14). In contrast, aggregating the entire inner cell mass of a human embryo with a mouse embryo would lead to a more widespread integration of the human cells, although it is unlikely such an organism could develop beyond a short time (Daylon et al. 2006).

Of most interest here are (1) interspecies chimeras where (2) one of the species is human, (3) the integration of cells is widespread, and (4) the integration involves reproductive cells or has the capacity to affect the germ line. This early interspecies research (ISR) would include, for example, injecting human ES cells into the blastocele (blastocyst cavity) of mouse or chicken embryos to study the properties of the ES cells as the animal embryo develops. The goal here would be to help assess the utility of human ES cells for eventual medical therapies (De Witt 2002; Committee on Guidelines 2005, 34; Shreeve 2005). If the embryos were to develop to birth, the resulting mouse or chicken would be an interspecies chimera containing "extensive and integrated cellular contributions from another species" (ISSCR 2006, 14). The cells would exist side by side but without integration of nuclear DNA between the two species (Committee on Guidelines 2005, 33).

Another potential chimera that has attracted attention is one in which human ES cells or their derivatives are transferred to nonhuman primates in a way that might significantly affect the central nervous system or the developing brain of the recipient animal (Brigid Hogan in Board on Life Sciences and Board on Health Sciences Policy 2004; Greene et al. 2005). Although intriguing, these interventions are noted only in passing here because they do not take place at the embryonic level, even though they may use human ES cells or their derivatives. This chapter touches on human-human, human-nonhuman, and nonhuman-human chimeras.

All have been proscribed by law in one or more nations and/or have been reviewed at least briefly by policy advisory committees. Although human-human chimeras are part of intra- rather than interspecies research, they evoke some of the same issues as interspecies chimeras.

CHIMERAS IN NATURE

Natural chimerism is a rare phenomenon that occurs within (but not between) species. For example fraternal twin cows are blood chimeras if, while they were fetuses, their circulatory systems were joined, blood was exchanged, and each was born with genetically distinct hematopoietic stem cells (Colorado State University n.d., 3). They are "trace" or "blood" chimeras because the tissue exchange is minimal and affects only the blood cells. A more complete form of chimerism occurs when two fertilized eggs (zygotes) fuse in an animal's uterus and the resulting offspring is tetragametic (has four parent cells). Similarly if a fertilized and an unfertilized egg combine, or a fertilized egg combines with two spermatozoa, the offspring will have three parent cells. The offspring in these cases would have cells from different gametes throughout the body (Schaub 2006, 30 n. 1). This phenomenon has been likened to stacking two jigsaw puzzles with different pictures and shaping them with the same cutter. If all the pieces are mixed, one can assemble a puzzle with parts from each picture (Chimera [genetics] n.d., 1). A chimera differs from a hybrid, where "every cell contains a mixture of genetic material from both originating species" (Mirkes 2006, 115–16). Signs of potential chimerism are an animal having eyes or fur of two different colors (Wood n.d.). Chimeras, which have mixed cells from two individuals, differ from hybrids, which have combined DNA from two different individuals in all of their body cells.

Chimeras also occur naturally in humans. Human fraternal twins who share the same placenta as fetuses will have a mixture of genetically distinct bone marrow cells (Genetic Mosaics n.d.). These twins are blood chimeras because the blood system is the only part of their body with two sets of genes. As a consequence they may also have two blood types. It is estimated that 8 percent of fraternal twins are blood chimeras (Wood n.d.). Occasionally in human development two fertilized eggs (zygotes) fuse to create a full chimera. If the zygotes are the same sex, no one may know of the chimerism unless blood tests have revealed the anomaly. If, however, one were a female and one a male, the child would have a mixture of XY and XX cells and would have intersex traits such as one testicle and one ovary. In one recent case a member of a pair of twins had ambiguous genitalia, and further tests revealed the twins were natural chimeras who shared only some of the genes inherited from their father. Physicians surmised that two sperm may have fused with the egg, "creating a cell with three sets of chromosomes which later split into two embryos having a normal complement of chromosomes." Alternatively the egg may have divided but not separated, leaving each cell to be fertilized by an individual spermatozoan (When Two Fuse with One 2007).

Chimerism in humans may not be detected if the zygotes are of the same sex and no anomalies are observed. In one case a fifty-two-year-old woman with three children was told, after tests to assess whether her children could be organ donors for her, that she could not be the mother of two of the children because they did not share her HLA haplotype. People usually inherit one HLA haplotype from each parent. This woman, however, had an unknown haplotype. Further inquiry, including tests of her brother, led doctors to speculate that two fertilized eggs had fused in her mother's uterus so she had cells in her body from four gametes. Such cases are thought to be very rare, with perhaps only thirty in the world today (Wood n.d.).

A variant of chimerism called microchimerism may be present to some extent in many people. Here a pregnant woman exchanges cells with her fetus and then carries the cells for years to come, affecting subsequent children (Schaub 2006, 30, n.1; Ainsworth 2003). If the exchange of cells takes place across generations, people might have cells in their bodies from their grandparents or siblings, making them what one writer calls "cellular mongrels" (Ainsworth 2003, 3). Tyler Hamilton, a renowned cyclist, tried in 2005 to use microchimerism as a defense against charges that he had used blood transfusions (Chimera on a Bike? 2005). When a test revealed that he had two types of blood cells, Hamilton said he was a chimera, and the different blood cells were the result of a "vanishing twin" rather than from any blood transfusion. The defense was diminished when his "minority cell population" dropped over a period of months, and geneticists pointed out that his minority cell population of 2 percent was more than he would have received from a previous fetus. As Hamilton wrote in his on-line journal, "If we've accomplished nothing else in this case, we have put a spotlight on the vanishing twin phenomenon" (Chimera on a Bike? 2005).

HUMAN-HUMAN CHIMERAS

What would be the rationale for creating a human chimera for research purposes by fusing human ES cells with human embryos? At present this question is not the subject of serious proposals to this author's knowledge, perhaps because the science has not progressed to a stage where such a creation would be useful, possible, or tenable. However, one can visualize a rationale for attempting this after what can be learned from transferring human ES cells to animal embryos has been exhausted. Knowledge gained from human-nonhuman transfer would logically lead to interest in testing the findings by fusing human ES cells with human embryos. Over twenty years ago members of the U.S. Human Embryo Research Panel (HERP), which was established to consider the ethical acceptability of various types of research involving embryos, mentioned in passing that human-human transfer could be engaged in for "lineage studies," to study gene therapy, or to prevent the symptoms of diseases such as cystic fibrosis by "seeding an embryo with one or more healthy cells" (Green 2001, 101).

Thinking about Dignity

The HERP categorized research involving embryos as ethically acceptable, warranting further review, or unacceptable for federal research funding. Research would fall into the "unacceptable" category were it to have potentially adverse effects on children, women, or men and should it fail to exercise respect due to the embryo. In addition, research raising "concern for public sensitivities about highly controversial research proposals" and "concern for the meaning of humanness, parenthood, and the succession of generations" could fall into that category (Green 2001, 100). Panel members also looked disfavorably on research having "very minor scientific or therapeutic value."

With these criteria in mind, the HERP briefly considered the ethics of human-human chimeras and deemed the development of such chimeras unacceptable for funding "with or without transfer." According to the panel the threat to human dignity was a central reason for deeming human-human chimeric research unacceptable for funding, but panel members did not elaborate on their reasoning. This leads one to question whether basic research creating a human-human chimeric embryo would violate human dignity in a way different from other types of research. Would the chimeric element make the intervention different from other nontherapeutic studies on human embryos? The HERP looked at the clinical use of human-human chimeras and regarded the transfer of human-human chimeras to a woman's uterus to be ethically unacceptable because it would offend "deeply held beliefs about individuation and personal identity" (National Institutes of Health 1994, 95). If one regards the embryo as having the moral status of a person, then by implication the individuality argument would apply to untransferred embryos too. According to this line of thought, fusing two human embryos or fusing one embryo with ES cells from another would intrude on the embryo's individuality and hence dignity.

This argument is predicated on the assumption that the human embryo has the moral status of a person, and it may not hold true without that assumption. Moreover, the preimplantation embryo does not necessarily have irreversible individuality in that it can still divide into two, three, four, or more embryos to yield a multiple pregnancy of identical twins, triplets, or quadruplets. The fourteen-day rule is in part predicated on the assumption that by fourteen days the embryo has passed the point where it could twin and is now destined to become a single individual. Similarly, fusion can occur before fourteen days. The potentiality for twinning or fusing means that individuality is not firmed until around fourteen days of development.

In addition, because chimeric fusions can occur in natural conditions to produce a single individual, it is hard to see how chimerism threatens individuality. An adult chimera is not two people in any legal or moral sense. He or she is simply a person with cells from two genomes in his or her body. Chimerism is part of the person's individuality. The same would apply for the embryo used in research. If the individuality of the person who is a natural chimera is not intruded upon, neither would it be for the embryo deliberately created to be a chimera for a short-term existence.

It is not, then, apparent how human-human chimerism itself is any more a violation of individuality and dignity than other studies in which embryos are examined and destroyed in the laboratory. One difference is that two embryos will be destroyed rather than one, unless existing ES cell lines are used. Moreover, individuality is a key value in our society. To act in a way that appears to intrude on it is to touch on a treasured value and to elicit understandable concerns. An alternative response to this dilemma is an appeal to the norms and regulations of embryo research, whereby human-human chimera studies would not be acceptable, at present at least, because no important rationales exist for the studies and because alternative ways of addressing questions about ES-cell development and function have not been exhausted. Researchers bear the burden of showing the need to use embryos; no evidence indicates that this burden has yet been met for human-human chimeras in laboratory research.

Thinking about Procreation

One objection to human-human chimeric research is that it would pave the way to clinical use such as transfer of a cleaving chimeric embryo to a woman's uterus for possible pregnancy and birth. Although such an action is highly remote, it is not altogether fanciful. In his book, *Remaking Eden*, Lee M. Silver presents a scenario of how a request for creating a human-human chimera might unfold (Silver 1997, 213–19). The basic scenario is presented here, with "facts" changed about the gender of the would-be parents and the simplicity of performing the act. In this version of the scenario, a gay male couple wants to have a child related to each of them with the help of an egg donor and surrogate.

The simplest method is for the couple to have two children, one sired by one of the men and the other sired by the second man. But this couple wants to have a child with a biological connection to both men. This could be achieved, conceivably, by retrieving eggs from a donor and fertilizing some with sperm from one partner and some with the sperm of the second. Only two embryos will be needed, one from each man. If the fertilizations are successful, the two cleaving embryos could be used to create a chimera, either by injecting ES cells from one embryo into a second recipient embryo or, in Silver's version, fusing intact cells from the two embryos. The resulting child would have cells from each partner. The mix would not be equal because cells from the recipient embryo would predominate over the ES cells from the donor embryo, but the goal of both men sharing biologically in one child would be met, at least in minute part.

The argument for this echoes justifications asserted for the other forms of collaborative reproduction—the desire of people who are infertile or who cannot conceive to have a child linked biologically to at least one potential parent; generally, this will be a genetic link. According to this argument, both fertile and infertile people have the same interests in reproducing biologically related children, although the infertile couple may need to use technological intervention. Infertility or the inability to have children for other reasons does not in itself mean a person lacks fundamental interests in procreation (Robertson 1994). A fundamental interest does not translate to an absolute interest, however, and limits on assisted reproductive technologies may be justifiable if the procedures would clearly harm offspring or are otherwise damaging. Would potential harm be so great in this case as to preclude this chimera scenario?

A strong case can be made that creating and transferring a human-human chimeric embryo for procreation would not at this point be ethical. First, there is no compelling reason to do this. Even if one accepts genetic relatedness as a legitimate goal, there is little nexus between this goal and a human-human chimera. Inserting ES cells from one embryo into the sphere of a recipient blastocyst would not achieve interrelatedness in a meaningful way. The child resulting from a person who contributed the full embryo would inherit mainly features of that dominant donor. It is not known how the cells from the ES-cell donor would be distributed; the child could be a strong or weak chimera, depending on how widespread the integration. The degree of chimerism would be greater if two intact embryos were fused rather than one embryo and one group of ES cells. Silver envisions the former technique, in which the zona pellucida of two embryos is dissolved and one embryo is "nudged" into the other (Silver 1997, 185). The new entity is given a new zona, and it subsequently divides as a single embryo.

Even if the degree of chimerism were strong, however, genetic relatedness would not be achieved. Cells, not genes, would mingle. Silver describes this for mouse models: "At the cellular level, nothing happens. Each individual cell retains its identity; no fusion between cells takes place. But, as the embryo develops, the cells derived from different parents mix together and communicate with each other as if they are all members of the same team. And when the animal is born, every tissue within it—including the brain and gonads—is a mixture of cells from the original two embryos" (Silver 1997, 179).

Second, the safety of the procedure obviously would be a concern (National Institutes of Health 1994, 43). If human-human chimeras are like animal-animal chimeras, the child might have blotchy skin reflecting the skin tone and textures of both contributing genomes. Moreover, if the embryos were of different sexes, the child could have intersex features and be born with reproductive anomalies that could cause emotional distress and prevent him or her from reproducing. Even if the embryos were of the same sex, however, the safety is questionable because of the difficulty of predicting how or whether the cells would be distributed through the body and what traits would result from this mosaic of cells.

Third, would human-human chimera use in reproduction threaten individuality? The answer here appears to be no. If only a limited number of ES cells were transferred, the cells from the ES cell donor might not affect the germ line or even the brain cells, making the procedure in some ways akin to tissue transplantation. With full embryo fusion, the interchange would be greater. In either case the child would remain a unique individual. His or her individuality would not be threatened any more than it would be from regular fertilization, unless we are oriented to thinking about a soul (for example, that combining two embryos would combine two souls). Once again, however, we would not say that a natural-born chimera possesses two souls, so it is not clear why a person who is a chimera by deliberate action would have two souls. Moreover, basing ethical arguments on beliefs about souls is not a useful framework for policymaking. Not only is it rooted in religion, but it fails to take into account different beliefs within and across religions.

Concerns about safety ground the deliberations in a more compelling and measurable dimension for policy purposes. The male partners' claim to procreate through human-human embryonic fusion on the whole is weak given the medical risks involved, absence of consensus about the procedure's ethics, and availability of reproductive alternatives for the two adults. Doing something risky for biological relatedness (and a dubious form of relatedness at that) and when alternatives exist pushes the adults' interests too far in relation to the physical well-being of a resulting child.

Policy Directions

Policy on human-human chimeras is sketchy. In the United States, the HERP, as discussed earlier, has judged it unacceptable for funding "with or without transfer." The report itself had little impact on policy, however, amid the panel's conclusion that embryos could ethically be created for research purposes and President Clinton's implicit rejection of this finding. The President's Council on Bioethics (PCB) recommended against human-human chimeras in various reports, and U.S. Senate Bill 1373 would have made it a crime to create or attempt to create a human chimera (defined as "beings with diverse human and non-human tissue") or to transport one in interstate commerce (U.S. Senate 2005b). The NAS Committee on Guidelines concluded that transferring ES cells "from any species" to human blastocysts should "not be permissible at this time" (Committee on Guidelines 2005).

The California Institute for Regenerative Medicine (CIRM) disallowed funding for "the introduction of any stem cells, whether human or non-human, into human embryos" (California Institute 2007, sec. 100030[d]). In a diffusion of policies, various embryonic stem cell research oversight committees (ESCROs) use the NAS language or modify it slightly. Canada's Assisted Human Reproduction Act of 2004 revolves around a licensing system for research. The act defines a chimera, in part, as an "embryo that consists of cells of more than one embryo, foetus or human being" (3b). It forbids creating this kind of chimera knowingly to create a human being (5-1-c) or for research purposes ("no person shall knowingly . . . create a chimera" [5-1-i]). The HFE Act of 2008 of the United Kingdom allows only a "permitted embryo" to be transferred to a woman. An embryo is not permitted if, among other things, it has had a cell "added to it other than by division of the embryo's own cells" (U.K. HFE Act 2008, Part 1.3(5)(4)(c)).

South Korea and Japan also explicitly forbid creating a child by fusing two human embryos. Taking a different stance, the International Society for Stem Cell Research (ISSCR) has accepted the insertion of human totipotent or pluripotent stem cells into human embryos up to fourteen days, provided the protocol was reviewed by a stem cell oversight committee or similar mechanism (ISSCR 2006, 7).

Existing regulations in the United States would presumably preclude transfer of human-human chimeras for procreation. The FDA, in a position that has generated differences of opinion, considers embryos that have been "more than minimally manipulated" to be cellular and tissue-based biological products that fall under the authority of the federal Food, Drug, and Cosmetics Act and the Public Health Service Act (Kopinsky 2004, 637). The FDA could assert its authority to regulate chimeras as biological products. Investigators seeking to transfer such embryos as part of clinical practice would need to submit an Investigational New Drug application. The FDA placed a clinical hold on ooplasm transfer for reproduction, thereby halting the practice, and it indicated it would do the same for reproductive cloning. Logically, it also would do the same for human-human chimeric embryos intended for procreation, provided its authority over embryos as biological products is legitimated. No focusing event elevates human-human chimeras to the status of a problem at this time. The use of human-human chimeras for procreation is not on the horizon in that it lacks technical feasibility and motivating rationale.

HUMAN-NONHUMAN CHIMERAS

Early interspecies chimeric research could involve injecting human ES cells into animal embryos or injecting animal ES cells into human embryos. Generally, when ES cells from one organism are fused with the embryo of another, the species of the recipient embryo will predominate. This section relates to the fusion of human ES cells with nonhuman embryos, or what some call human-nonhuman interspecifics (HNHIs).

Cell transfers can be accomplished by aggregating two embryos or by injecting individual or clumps of ES cells from one embryo into a genetically distinct recipient embryo (Roussant 2004, xxii; Daylon et al. 2006). Fusing two zygotes or early-stage embryos is the opposite of twinning, where an embryo divides into two separate but identical twins (Genetic Mosaics n.d.). The fusion can take place within the same species or across species. The cells will keep their character, so the organism will have tissues from two or more organisms side by side (Singleton 2000, 1088). Whereas hybrids have DNA from two parents in every cell, a chimera, with genetically distinct cells from two different embryos, will have mixed cells from four genetic parents in its system.

Researchers first reported creating a chimeric mouse in 1968 when they inserted an ES cell from one mouse embryo into a three- to five-day embryo of a second (Gardner 1968). In transgenic mouse research today investigators generally transfer eight to twelve ES cells from one mouse embryo to the center of a second five- to seven-day mouse embryo (blastocyst). It is believed that only a limited number of cells actually contribute to the developing embryo; the number depends in part on the quality of the cells. Whether only a few cells or the entire inner cell mass is inserted depends on the research question. The resulting mouse will have cells from four genetically distinct parents in its system and will have a mosaic quality. For example, ES cells from a mouse embryo with parents having black fur (one set of parents) may be fused with the embryo with parents having white fur (a second set of parents) (Genetic Mosaics n.d.). After gestation in a surrogate mouse, a chimeric (tetraparental) mouse will be born with cells from each set of parents and with mottled fur of black and white. Coat color is usually the measure used to assess the degree of chimerism, which can be tailored by investigators. Varying the number of cells transferred to the recipient embryo affects the characteristics of the offspring (U.K. Department of Health 2007b, Appendix B. 1.3.4). (See Fig. 1.1)

Mice and other rodents are commonly used to create intraspecies chimeras as a method in the study of the course and treatment of human disease by use of a knockout technique. The goal is to create a line of mice lacking the gene associated with a given human disease in order to study ways of treating and understanding mechanisms of the disease. In the knockout method researchers delete a gene from mouse ES cells, locate those cells with the inactivated gene, and then inject the cells into a recipient mouse embryo (Nuffield Council on Bioethics 2005, 5.19–5.20). The resulting mouse is a chimera with normal cells from one set of parents and some cells with the inactivated gene from the second set of parents. Mice whose germ cells pick up modified cells are "founder mice" and are

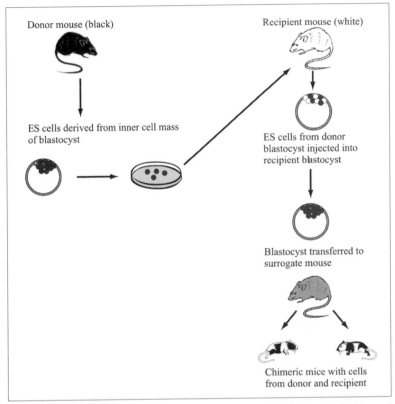

Figure 1.1.   A Method for Obtaining Intraspecies Chimeras for Research. Adapted from http://www.biotechnology4u.com/animal_biotechnology_ stem_cell_technology.html. Accessed December 5, 2008.

bred so that the altered gene gets into the germ line. The last step works only some of the time, so chimeric mice are bred over several generations to secure a stable line of mice with the mutation (Travis 1992). These would be transgenic mice derived from chimeras.

Similar fusion techniques are used between animal species to create interspecies chimeras. For example, mouse ES cells can be made to differentiate to neuronal stem cells, which are precursors of motor neurons. These cells are then injected into chicken embryos to test whether they function as they are supposed to do (Committee on Guidelines 2005). These studies indicate whether the cells differentiate and whether they

can be controlled so as not to form tumors (Pollack 2006). A second species, the chicken, is used because chicken eggs can be monitored closely.
A hole can be cut into the eggshell to observe development, whereas this
cannot be done for the mouse. In another example ES cells from dogs
can be transferred to mouse blastocysts to examine their functioning.
Dogs can serve as better models for human diseases than mice, but it is
harder to control their reproductive cycles, so canine ES cells are used
for pragmatic reasons.

Interspecies chimeras of interest here are those in which one of the
species providing or receiving ES cells or their derivatives is human. If it
is in the human-nonhuman direction, this involves transferring human
ES cells or their derivatives to animals at different levels of development
(embryo, fetal, neonate). Alternatively, adult stem cells may be transferred
to a fetal or adult animal, which would produce a trace chimera with limited numbers of human cells in its body (Committee on Guidelines 2005,
34). Constructing an organ from human stem cells and then transferring
it to an animal to test for safety and efficacy would be such a case.

Transferring human ES cells or their derivatives to mouse embryos
enables examination of the potential of human ES cells to differentiate
and become functional tissues within living organisms (Svendsen 2006).
For example, if investigators could direct human ES cells to differentiate
to insulin-producing cells, theoretically these cells could be injected into
patients with type 1 diabetes to replace the cells destroyed by the impact of
the disease. But before clinical trials can proceed, safety and efficacy must
be established in preclinical testing with animal models. Mouse recipients would enable investigators to ask: Will the recipient's body reject the
cells? Will the recipient's body destroy the new cells as it did the original
cells because of the underlying diabetes? Will the cells work properly by
adjusting their production of insulin when glucose levels change in the
body? (Pollack 2006).

One team of investigators reported they had transferred human
ES cells to mouse embryos by two techniques and demonstrated that
the human cells could engraft, proliferate, and differentiate; their data
"demonstrate[d] the feasibility of this approach, using mouse embryos
as a surrogate for [human ES-cell] differentiation" (Daylon et al. 2006,
90). They also described investigations by other researchers in which (1)

human ES cells injected into a chick embryo "were shown to proliferate and contribute to neural cell types" and (2) human ES cells injected into the brains of fetal mice "gave rise to functional human neurons within the adult mouse brain."

The authors of the latter study report that their investigation demonstrated that human ES cells can "differentiate into authentic human neurons in vivo" (Muotri et al. 2005). This creates a model for studying how and to what extent human ES cells can differentiate and migrate in a living system. Chimeras could facilitate the investigation into other matters such as how the cells function over time and how they respond to signals in the host organism. The same authors assert that if undifferentiated human ES cells are injected into the brain of a rat model for Parkinson's disease and survive, they "can be used as long-term carriers of therapeutic gene products" (Muotri et al. 2005). They further assert that human ES cells can be genetically manipulated and then injected into a mouse brain to produce a "mouse-human chimeric nervous system" on which potential therapies can be tested over a long period of time.

Transferring human adult stem cells to animal recipients is common practice. Researchers disagree, however, on the need for studies using human ES cells. Some claim the studies are not supported by strong scientific rationales and that other methods can be used to test the potential of ES cells or their derivatives (Board on Life Sciences and Board on Health Sciences Policy 2004). Others, however, are persuaded it is necessary. Policymakers in the United Kingdom, for example, see "huge benefits" if the creation of chimeras and cybrids yields information about human ES cells and promotes medical therapies (U.K. House of Commons 2007, 47, 49).

Additional considerations are whether and to what extent such research will include higher-order species. Some researchers regard human-mouse chimeras as having limited use because human cells would die off and be lost (United Kingdom. Parliament 2007a). They argue that human-nonhuman monkey chimeras might yield more useful information about the abilities of human ES cells and their potential for forming tumors (Committee on Guidelines 2005, 34). A different envisioned line of chimeric research is to inject large numbers of human neural cells into the brains of species closer to humans such as the Rhesus monkey to study human neurons in a living brain (Greene et al. 2005). A goal would be to create a living model to study the structure and function of human neurons, especially in relation to disease and the testing of drugs (Cheshire 2007, 49). The research would examine the extent to which various kinds of neurons could help treat spinal cord injuries or degenerative diseases (Committee on Guidelines 2005, 33).

Thinking about Dignity

In what ways, if any, would research involving HNHIs violate human dignity? If only a small number of differentiated human stem cells were transferred to a mouse embryo, this would result in a weak chimeric mouse with a scattering of human cells existing alongside its own cells. More significant mingling might raise more objections, as in transferring large numbers of human neuronal cells to the brains of mice that have a genetic disorder that causes all the neurons in their cerebellums to die (Cohen 2007b, 127). Transferring human neurons to mouse brains just before neuronal death would enable study of the functioning of the human cells. A concern has been raised that ISR will be used to transfer human neurons to nonhuman brains in numbers that will cause the mouse to take on human-like levels of cognition, perception, or consciousness (Board on Life Sciences and Board on Health Sciences Policy 2004, 7).

Cynthia Cohen regards objections to extensive chimerism based on the claim the studies would harm human dignity as the most persuasive of criticisms raised against this research (Cohen 2007b). Defining dignity as a cluster of capacities of humans that "render them worthy of respect," she links objections based on human dignity to the possibility the resulting animal might have human capacities that it will not be able to exercise (Cohen 2007b, 125; see also Karpowicz, Cohen, and van der Kooy 2005). If "certain human bodily components" appear in human-nonhuman chimeric beings, these capacities "would be severely restricted in their exercise or even destroyed" (Cohen 2007b, 126). An animal with an extensive human-like brain would violate human dignity "because it would render the resulting chimera incapable of exercising its distinctively human capacities, since its brain would be imprisoned in an animal-like body" (126). The same principle would apply if a chimera were created by injecting large amounts of undifferentiated human ES cells into an animal embryo and the cells migrated to the brain in a way that would lead to a chimera with a "human brain" (126). The concern is that human-like characteristics in animals would be an affront to what is uniquely human.

Johnston and Eliot also regard the human dignity argument as a reasonable objection to the creation of chimeras. Having in mind blended beings, they conclude human dignity would be violated if life is cruel for the chimera, assuming it has human elements that cannot be exercised when its life involves being a subject for medical research. Dignity would be violated too by allowing individuals or institutions to "intentionally creat[e] compromised human beings or part-human beings" and to use these beings as a means to another's end (Johnston and Eliot 2003, 2). In short, these authors look to a postnatal adult being (not an embryo or a fetus) to assert the dignity argument.

Although the creation of and research on beings with human and nonhuman traits may be valid concerns with nonhuman primates, this dignity-based objection holds less weight in research involving rodents and other animals. Here the transfer of neural cells, for example, is not likely to lead to human-like cognition. Among other things the human brain is infinitely more complex than a mouse brain: "It is more than the cellular components that make a human brain. It's the connections, the blood vessels that feed them; it's the various surfaces on which they migrate, the timing by which various synaptic molecules are released and impact other things, like molecules from the bloodstream and from the bone" (Shreeve 2005, 47).

Nao Kobayashi notes that it is confusing to create images of "a bit of man in a mouse brain," especially since early research showed that only some human stem cells survive when transferred to a mouse brain (Kobayashi 2003). Even if human cells were to survive to affect the mouse brain, the vastly different brain structures between humans and mice make it untenable to expect mice to take on cognitive abilities resembling those of humans. Brain size gives another reason for supposing this. A mouse with large numbers of human cells in its brain would need a large head for the brain to have human functions (Karpowicz 2003), when in fact the mouse brain has one-thousandth the number of neurons as a human brain (Cheshire 2007, 50). It might even be possible to produce a mouse brain "composed entirely of human cells," but this does not mean it is a human brain (Greely et al. 2007, 32). Moreover, it is not clear how this could be an affront to humanity.

Observers differ about whether transferring human neurons to mouse brains is equivalent to "conferring humanity" on mice. The claim in itself may help explain public reaction to such studies (Rollin 2007a, 56). To some, such studies could confer an attribute of humans onto mice (Lavieri 2007) or eventually could create a mouse with human neurons that will "surprise the researcher by exhibiting behavior suggestive of higher levels of awareness" and, consequently, necessitate caution (Cheshire 2007, 49). To others the idea of a mouse with observable human traits is a "hyperbolic misnomer" (Rollin 2007a, 57).

Vast differences between rodents and primates make the transfer of undifferentiated or differentiated human ES cells to developing rodents for short lives a different issue from that of the transfer of significant numbers of neural cells to primates. As pointed out by DeGrazia, studies transferring human ES cells or neural stem cells to higher-level primates are more significant than those using rodents as recipients because the former have "relatively large craniums." The "long brain-development time seems more conducive to the development of humanlike brains than in the case of other lab animals" (DeGrazia 2007, 310). In the case of either rodents or primates, however, it is not clear how the studies would harm human dignity. To DeGrazia "concerns about human dignity prove insignificant" (309). Among other things, it is unrealistic to consider that rodents would have "achieved the cognitive complexity of, say, a borderline person or person" with full moral status. Even if cognition were affected, the dignity of humans would not be threatened by having more "individuals with full moral status" (326). At issue is the interest of the being itself: It is wrong to bring a being into the world who is "unlikely to enjoy the social supports that such a being deserves."

Thinking about Procreation

As noted above, an objection to human-nonhuman ISR is that it will lead to the creation of beings with both human and nonhuman features. The presumption is that people will be so drawn to the science that they will not want or be able to create boundaries, and the resulting beings will look like or be like humans.

In a scientific sense it is unrealistic to assume the birth of mixed human-nonhuman beings that look or act like human beings. First, it is unlikely that fusing entire cell masses of human and mouse embryos would yield a developing fetus, much less an organism that would survive to birth. Second, even if the resultant organism did survive, it is unknown whether human cells would still be present in such numbers and types as to produce a being with human and nonhuman traits. Investigations to date that have introduced human ES cells to animal embryos have been "very unimpressive," according to one source, particularly because human embryos develop more slowly and follow a different pattern, which means the human cells are lost early in development (U.K. Parliament 2007a). Daylon et al. (2006, 7) found that mouse chimeras could implant in surrogate mice but that the human ES cells "seemed to disrupt embryogenesis in most cases." The potential of a human-animal being with extensive chimerism is remote for distant species; investigators predict it is unlikely that human-mouse chimeras would develop into viable chimeric embryos. The likelihood of a mouse with human-like thinking is exceedingly remote. It is not known whether the transfer of significant numbers of human neural cells would enhance cognition in more closely related recipient primates (Greene et al. 2005).

Another matter is how one determines which human traits would be problematic if they appeared in animals. For example, mice have been modeled by gene knockout technology to lack the ability to produce certain proteins, and this results in their having cystic fibrosis. These mice have a pervasive "human" presence because they have been engineered to have the equivalent of a human disease. Yet far from being targeted as unethical, the creation of mouse models for a range of human diseases is a sought-after goal. A disease, therefore, is not regarded as a human attribute to be avoided in animals.

Some suggest that the presence of observable human-like features in an animal would matter. In PCB hearings, William Hurlbut observed that dignity is "not just a matter of function" and that human dignity is preserved by "preserving the uniqueness of the human form" (President's Council on Bioethics 2005c, 17). According to Robert and Baylis, chimeras provoke moral confusion only if tangible evidence of the crossing of species exists (Robert and Baylis 2003). Karpowicz responds that as long as humans and animals are recognizable as humans and animals, there will not be moral confusion (Karpowicz 2003).

The appearance criterion has failings however. What if, to use a fanciful example, a mouse's paw is genetically modified to have appendages that resembled human fingers? This would be problematic under the human-features visual test. But would a mouse with its paw digits modified through transgenics to resemble human fingers—a cosmetic and external change—be significantly more human-like than a mouse modeled to have cystic fibrosis, a human disease that affects its entire biological system? Or, consider the chimpanzee Washoe, who died at age 42 in 2007, taking with her an impressive English vocabulary. Trained in American Sign Language, she was the first nonhuman to learn a human language (Friends of Washoe n.d.). By intensive training rather than a biological intervention, Washoe took on human-like language and was regarded with fascination rather than repulsion.

In the end, policy advisory groups seem more drawn to issues raised by the transfer of neural cells to primates rather than to rodents. A working group from the Phoebe R. Berman Bioethics Institute at Johns Hopkins University, for one, recommended that human-to-nonhuman primate neural grafting be done only with special review requiring investigators "wherever possible, to look for and report changes in cognitive function," especially in the area of the brain affected by the grafting (Greene et al. 2005). Acknowledging that human-nonhuman neural grafting could result in suffering of a cognitively enhanced animal, the group advised oversight committees to be especially attuned to the "proportion of engrafted human cells," the "stage of neural development," the closeness of the species brain size to that of humans, and the closeness of the targeted area of the brain between humans and the recipient species (386). The NAS Committee on Guidelines recommended not proceeding with research in which human ES cells are injected into nonhuman primate blastocysts, as did the NIH in its 2009 guidelines (Committee on Guidelines 2005; National Institutes of Health 2009).

Other policy advisory groups and scholars have proposed a precautionary approach to chimeric research that is applicable to all species.

Karpowicz et al., for example, propose transferring the smallest number of cells possible to an embryo, using only species not closely related to humans, and using dissociated (individual) stem cells rather than the whole inner cell mass (Karpowicz, Cohen, and van der Kooy 2005, 127). The number of cells could gradually be increased over time if no "human-like structure" appeared during neural development in preliminary studies (Cohen 2007b, 135).

Thinking about Species

A fairly extensive body of literature has developed about the relation between human-nonhuman chimeric research and thinking about species. In a lead article for a symposium in the *American Journal of Bioethics* about NHNIs, Robert and Baylis looked at reasons for finding human-nonhuman chimeras objectionable and concluded that the "most plausible objection" is that the studies could cause moral confusion about species boundaries (Robert and Baylis 2003). The authors argued that fixed lines between species do not exist in the scientific sense but that people believe they do and make "everyday moral decisions on the basis of this belief" (6). The moral status of humans is fixed, but the status of animals depends on the relationship that exists between them and humans (9). Humans "attach considerable symbolic importance to classificatory systems and actively shun anomalous practices that threaten cherished boundaries" (7).

If a chimera were developed with observable interspecies features, Baylis and Robert argue, it would leave people "baffled" and "fearful" if they did not know whether the being was human or what their responsibilities would be toward the being (8). The authors did not advocate prohibiting human-nonhuman chimeras, but they acknowledged a societal concern in preserving "boundaries between human and nonhuman animals" (10–11). Before chimeric research leading to "the creation of new creatures for whom there is no apparent a priori moral status" proceeds, humans must figure out their commitments to humans and nonhumans alike (11).

Some of the essayists who responded to the symposium article questioned whether moral confusion was a valid objection to human-nonhuman chimeras. Mark Sagoff discerned a gap between vision and reality; the chimeras proposed today (entities destroyed early in development) were far less confusing than the speculative type of chimeras contemplated by Robert and Baylis (Sagoff 2003, 30). In fact, he continued, the examples of proposed research they gave were not "morally problematic" in the sense of confusing the lines between humans and nonhumans (31).

Phillip Karpowicz challenged Robert and Baylis to give examples of ongoing chimeric research in which human traits actually appear along with nonhuman traits (Karpowicz 2003). Hilary Bok also disputed the likelihood of confusion, stating that most chimeras (with the exception of one caused by transfer of "substantial numbers of human neural cells into a nonhuman embryo") would not be confusing. She also regarded moral confusion to be a weak objection; on the contrary, confusion could encourage a reexamination of current ways of thinking (Bok 2003, 26). Andrew W. Siegel made a similar point: confusion can helpfully "[mark] a stage in the process of moral evolution" (Siegel 2003, 3).

To Rollin, confusion would allow an opportunity to question species as an unchanging concept and to modify assumptions. If species are indeterminate, he wrote, "we cannot tell with any exactitude where one species begins and another ends," including humans (Rollin 2003, 15). This supposedly "fixed moral category" between human and nonhuman species might better be rendered flexible, especially if it leads to improvement in the well-being of members of nonhuman species (see also Robert and Baylis 2003). David Castle thought any confusion would be "the embodiment of the clash between the absolute moral status of human beings qua human beings and the conditional moral status of other organisms." Combining the two (by creating adult beings) is like "mixing the oil and water of fundamental moral intuitions" (Castle 2003, 28). A reasonable response is to regard beings as "organisms in their own right," irrespective of their species (29). Henry Greely thought it more pertinent to object to chimeras created for "entertainment or 'art'" than for medical purposes (Greely 2003, 19). All novel organisms can be objectionable; the chimeric technique is not the deciding factor.

In these and other essays scholars have looked to the interests of the beings created through chimeric techniques. Streiffer, for example, asked, "Under what circumstances, if any, would the introduction of human material render an animal the moral equivalent of a normal human adult ('enhance the animal's moral status')?" Second, "under what circumstances, if any, is it morally permissible to enhance an animal's moral status?" (Streiffer 2006; see also Streiffer 2005).

Streiffer concluded that a status enhancement could be a benefit, but this could be done only if "there are reasonable assurances in place that its new moral status will be adequately respected" (Streiffer 2006, 5). To be avoided is "a situation in which a transplant of human material into a developing animal renders the animal the moral equivalent of a normal adult human . . . and the animal continues being treated as animals are usually treated in biomedical research" (6). Because protecting a higher moral status for the animal would be "incompatible with the research objectives which motivated the use of an animal to begin with," in most cases, "status-enhancing research is unethical" (7). If the intervention would enhance the animal's moral status, investigators should either stop development at the embryonic stage or not introduce significant numbers of human ES cells into the animal embryo in the first place (Streiffer 2005, 348).

Another dimension of animals' interests in chimeric research relates to the proliferation of animals needed to receive ES cells, provide eggs, or serve as surrogates. By one estimate, up to 150–175 blastocysts must be injected with mouse ES cells to yield one mouse-mouse chimera for transgenic research (Animal Testing 2006). From this process thirty to fifty mice will be born with the different skin colors that indicate a successful fusion, and of these mice two to six will have skin and hair traits indicating 70 percent or greater ES-cell contribution. This figure indicates "a good chance for embryonic stem cell contribution to the germ line." Procuring eggs and embryos means mice are superovulated (unless eggs are procured from a slaughterhouse) and mated. The fertilized eggs are then collected after death from smaller animals or by surgical extraction from larger animals (Boyd Group 1999, 7). These burdens for research animals are not unique to research involving chimeras.

Although most chimeric organisms are killed as embryos, fetuses, or neonates, when they have little or no consciousness, some will presumably develop to adulthood, including those in complex species. It is not known whether these chimeras would face discomforts, seizures, or distress beyond those associated with being research animals. Brigid Hogan cautioned that if human cells were "functionally incorporated" into the developing brain or germ line of nonhuman embryos or fetuses that then developed to birth and adulthood, this manipulation could cause "distress to the nonhuman recipient by disruption of its innate behavioral traits, sensitivity to environmental cues or drugs, circadian rhythm, breeding cycle, and its general 'sense of well-being'" (Board on Life Sciences and Board on Health Sciences Policy 2004).

Diana Schaub suggested that fully chimeric animals (not those with just a few cells from another species) may not feel at ease if the character of the species has been affected (President's Council on Bioethics 2005c, 2). Although little evidence pertains to this, it is possible that harboring cells from another species could have unsettling effects. In a widely publicized case of chimerism, a geep created by the fusion of early-stage embryos from a goat and a sheep was born in 1984 (Fehilly, Willadsen, and Tucker 1984). The geep had an odd appearance, with hairy goat and woolly sheep patches arising in a "hodgepodge" fashion on its coat representing two genetically distinct sets of cells (Colorado State University n.d.; Schaub 2006, 34). Its creator, Steen Willadsen, observed: "The animal behaved like a goat, but did not quite smell like one, and preferred the company of sheep. Its sheep cells were male but the sex of its goat cells was not known. It proved fertile in many matings with ewes [female sheep] but has not, so far, with does [female goats]" (Silver 2006, 181).

Policy Directions

Policy on human-nonhuman chimeric research is more developed than that for other types of early ISR. In Anglo-American countries, for example, Canada and the United Kingdom have detailed licensing structures. Canada's policy, based on the Assisted Human Reproduction Act and on stem-cell guidelines of Canada's Institutes of Health Research (Baylis and Robert 2007, 42), disallows the creation of human-human or human-nonhuman chimeras. Under these rules, human ES cells cannot be fused with human or nonhuman embryos or with fetuses. The rules prohibit the transfer of (1) human or nonhuman ES cells to a human embryo, (2) human or nonhuman ES cells to a human fetus, (3) human ES cells to a nonhuman embryo, or (4) human ES cells to a nonhuman fetus (Canadian Institutes of Health Research 2006, 42). The rules apply to investigators using federal funding, but they are inclusive because no privately funded research using human ES cells is ongoing in Canada.

The United Kingdom's HFE Act 2008 forbids an "admixed embryo" from being transferred to a woman. One type of admixed embryo is a "human embryo that has been altered by the introduction of one or more animal cells," which is a chimera (U.K. HFE Act 2008, Part 1.4(6)(d)). In Australia, the Prohibition of Human Cloning for Reproduction and the Regulation of Human Embryo Research Amendment Act 2006 forbids creating a human-nonhuman chimeric embryo. Internationally, the ISSCR approves the transfer of human ES cells to animals at any stage of development—embryos, fetuses, or adults—to create chimeric animals, provided the proposal passes extra review (ISSCR 2006, 7). It advised extra review to avoid chimerism in the germ line or cerebral cortex, which could happen if the chimerism took place early in development and the cells were widely integrated into the developing animal. To avoid the remote possibility of human-like characteristics developing with species close to humans, the ISSCR advises extra review before transferring human cells to nonhuman primates (7).

In the United States, as discussed in the Introduction, the Committee on Guidelines recommended a heightened oversight plan in which the transfer of human ES cells or their derivatives to nonhuman animals "at any stage of embryonic, fetal, or postnatal development" would be permissible but only after notification, review, and approval by an ES-cell oversight ESCRO committee (Committee on Guidelines 2005, 4). The Committee on Guidelines advised investigators to be alert to the possibility of the animals taking on human traits or appearance (Committee on Guidelines 2005, 41) and to monitor the transmission of human ES cells to see which organs are affected by the migration of cells through the body.

In his presentation to the Committee on Guidelines, Greely proposed a tiered review procedure to address the concern that nonhuman species will carry human traits. To Greely, much human-nonhuman chimeric research is standard and does not need heightened review. If, however, there is a "non-trivial chance" of conferring "significant aspects of humanness on nonhuman organisms," he recommended that research must be preceded by "specific and detailed discussion of the ethical issues involved in such work" in an IRB or similar body (Board on Life Sciences and Board on Health Sciences Policy 2004, 10). If a study fails the review, it can be controlled or forbidden, but otherwise regulation should be minimal (14). Greely also accepted heightened review before allowing human-nonhuman chimeras to mate if there is "any barely plausible chance of creating gametes with a diploid human genome" that could lead to the "fertilization of or by the 'human gamete.'"

Another venue for guidelines for human-nonhuman chimeras occurred at Stanford University, where Irving Weissman in 2000 shared ideas with colleagues about various experiments involving chimeras he was considering. In one he proposed transferring human neuronal stem cells from aborted fetuses that had been donated for research to the brains of fetal mice that had been altered to lose nearly all their neurons shortly before birth (Greely et al. 2007, 27). Weismann's idea was to transfer the human neurons into the fetal brains just before the intrinsic neurons of the subject mice died. The resulting mice would be models for studying how human neurons functioned in a living system and how they differentiated and migrated. The mice would also have been altered to have severe combined immunodeficiency so they would not reject the cells (31). The goal was for the cells to differentiate and migrate. Some mice would be aborted, and their brains studied at autopsy, and others would be born before their brains were autopsied. Still others would live as "laboratory animal[s] that could be used for experiments on living, in vivo, human neurons" (31). The work would "create a living model in which to investigate the aggregate structure and complex function of human neurons and their susceptibility to disease, drugs and toxins" (Cheshire 2007, 49).

To explore the issues associated with this and related studies, a working group was formed at the university, which concluded in 2002 that the experiments would be ethically acceptable within limits. For technical reasons Weissman did not conduct the experiments, but the report was revised and published in 2007 along with invited essays (Greely et al. 2007). The publication can be considered part of the varied guidelines for chimeric research that are emerging, even though it is advisory only. Its authors recommended that (1) proper procedures be followed to secure the human cells, (2) studies be carried out "in stages" and with careful monitoring for out-of-the-ordinary behaviors in mice or the appearance of "human-like structures in the mouse brains," (3) information about the studies be made known to the public, and (4) the mice not be allowed to breed in the unlikely event human gametes ever formed from the human neuronal stem cells (37). The Committee on Guidelines also deemed it not permissible at this time to "[breed] animals in which human embryonic stem cells have been introduced at any stage of development" (Committee on Guidelines 2005, 108). The NIH guidelines make ineligible for funding the breeding of animals if the addition of human ES or iPS cells "may contribute to the germ line" (National Institutes of Health 2009).

Policy relating to chimeras is flexible in the United States with similar recommendations issuing from the NAS, CIRM, ISSCR, and ESCROs. These recommendations generally (1) distinguish among three categories of research (not needing ESCRO review, needing ESCRO review, and not permissible at this time), (2) recommend against breeding human-nonhuman chimeras, and (3) urge caution in studies involving nonhuman primates. The recommended guidelines are decentralized in that local ESCROs can develop their own oversight policies, and there is some evidence of a diffusion of policies across ESCROs. Robert and Baylis see the report and the U.S. system as "strikingly liberal" (2005, 15). Although in some ways the guidelines are permissive, in other ways they are more cautious than might be expected. In light of the absence of extended deliberations and carefully constructed rationales for limiting chimeric research (especially in nonbreeding animals), for example, the recommendations are preemptive.

NONHUMAN-HUMAN CHIMERAS

Would it be ethically acceptable to transfer animal ES cells to human embryos for research purposes? At present there is no rationale to do so. As representatives of the Wellcome Trust put it, "It is hard to envisage any scientist applying to put mouse embryonic stem cells into a human embryo; there would be no point" (United Kingdom. Parliament 2007a). Yet provisions are included in various policies; for example, Canada's Institutes of Health Research bar research in which nonhuman ES cells are transferred to a human embryo or fetus (Canadian Institutes of Health Research 2006, 42).

For the sake of argument, assume that two studies with equivalent scientific justifications are proposed. They are similar in intent and method but have one difference: in Study A investigators will introduce animal ES cells into a human embryo, whereas in Study B they will introduce human ES cells into a human embryo. Both studies meet informed consent and other principles for ethical research using embryos. Assuming that human-human research chimeras do not in themselves violate human dignity as long as norms are followed, would the animal ES cells in Study A render the research a greater intrusion on human dignity than the human ES cells in Study B? Does the presence of animal cells make a qualitative difference? The Christian Medical Fellowship in the United Kingdom holds that it does: "Humans have an innate dignity absent from the animal kingdom, and there is a rich meaning to being human. Deliberately blurring the fundamental barrier between humans and non-human animals by admixing genetic material in the same embryo blurs boundaries, offends the dignity of us all, and risks changing the future of all mankind" (United Kingdom. Parliament 2007j).

If this is one's basic supposition, fusing animal cells with human embryos does indeed violate human dignity because this combines material from a less-regarded species with that of the more highly regarded human. But if this is not one's basic supposition, it is unclear how the presence of animal cells would be a greater affront to human dignity when the embryo is destroyed after investigation and is not used for procreation. One response is that the human embryo is accorded a higher moral status than an animal embryo of any species and ought to be protected for its inherent value, even when it is used in research. Yet again, it is not clear why the mere presence of animal cells renders the study unacceptable if the intent and outcome of studies A and B are the same. A more persuasive line of argument to prevent Study B is to rely on the norms and principles of embryo research. For example have investigators met their burden of demonstrating the worthiness of their research? Have they exhausted less intrusive alternatives? Are the studies likely to produce important scientific or clinical information? If transferring animal cells to human embryos does not meet these expectations, the investigation would be unsupportable.

SUMMARY

Intraspecies and interspecies chimeric procedures are widely practiced in research without appreciable ethical or policy concern (Board on Life Sciences and Board on Health Sciences Policy 2004, 1). When they are created as part of the study of human ES cells, and when one of the species is human, however, chimeras have attracted more attention. The degree of concern varies by several factors including the biological matter mixed, the relation between the organisms mixed, the stage of development at which the mixing takes place, and whether the fusion occurs naturally or though human intervention (Greely 2003, 17–18).

Various publicized events in the early 2000s triggered discussions about interspecies animal chimeras. These included the births of a chimeric "geep" (goat cell masses to sheep embryos) and a chick/quail (a quail that cheeped like a chick after the transfer of brain cells to chick embryos (Cohen 2007b, 131). These oddities conveyed the message that ISR on chimeras could produce odd and observable changes in offspring. Advances in the isolation and derivation of human ES cells in the same time period drew attention to the possibility of testing human ES cells in vivo by creating short-term human-nonhuman chimeras in a range of combinations, including transferring a small number of human ES cells to mouse embryos and transferring large numbers of human neural cells to fetal mouse brains (Greely et al. 2007). Various reports on the ethics of and guidelines for HNHIs were written and disseminated in the United States, the United Kingdom, Canada, and other countries.

If deliberations about chimeras have unfolded incrementally, so have resulting policies. A default policy apparatus is in play in the United States with recommendations to proceed cautiously. The ad hoc ethics committee at Stanford University, for example, accepted human-nonhuman ISR but recommended stopping research if odd behaviors occurred or human-like structures were detected in the recipient animal's brain (Cohen 2007a; Greely et al. 2007, 37). Karpowicz, Cohen, and van der Kooy proposed the following, whereby investigators should "(1) limit the number of stem cells transferred to the animal to the smallest number necessary to reach reliable scientific conclusions; (2) choose a host animal that is not closely related, either structurally or functionally, to humans; and (3) transfer only dissociated human neural stem cells, rather than whole masses of organized tissue, to prenatal nonhuman hosts" (Cohen 2007b, 132).

Cohen endorsed a similar step-by-step approach in transferring human neural cells to nonhuman brains: gradually increase the number of cells and gradually expand the area of the affected recipient brain (Cohen 2007b, 132). In this approach experiments move by degrees and would be halted if problems arose (Baylis and Robert 2007, 44; Greely et al. 2007, 37).

Several observations can be made about the weight of objections raised for human-nonhuman chimera research. First, human-human chimeric research is not a live policy problem at present. The fusion of human embryos for research purposes does not appear to be practiced in the research setting if the absence of published reports is a guide. In the event that it proceeds, evidence is not available that human-human fusion for laboratory research is so distinguishable from other techniques as to require regulations beyond the norms and principles of research using embryos in general.

Fusing human embryos (or human ES cells with human embryos) is arguably not a greater affront to human dignity than other techniques, assuming equally valid purposes of the studies. Nor is the objection compelling that this technique should be treated differently because clinicians might be tempted to try it for procreation. Human-human chimeras are not a supportable addition to fertility treatment. Even if demand developed, the technique would likely follow the path of twinning, cytoplasmic transfer, and nuclear transfer, which are novel possibilities on hold because of uncertain safety and the absence of a consensus about their ethical acceptability.

Second, issues relating to human-nonhuman chimeras do not pose substantial ethical challenges based on human dignity, temptation to use for procreation, and blurring of species lines. The bulk of the research involves transfer of a small number of human cells to prenatal or postnatal rodents or other distant species. It is unpersuasive to assert that transferring human cells to rodents is an affront to human dignity any more than it is to assert that culturing human ES cells on animal feeder cells is an affront. To inject human cells into a living animal at the pre- or postnatal level does not in itself tip the scales to harm dignity.

Even the transfer of human ES-cell-derived neural cells to mouse brains lacks the hallmarks of a "problem." If such a transfer were to lead to cognitive changes, it would have more of an impact on the mouse's welfare than on human dignity. Human cells in a mouse brain do not make a "man in the mouse," as Kobayashi put it. It is more accurate to think of mice with "human DNA sequences or cells/tissues" than of a "humanized mouse" (Kobayashi 2003).

Transferring large numbers of human ES cells or their derivatives to primates is more complex in light of greater research protections for primates than for other animals and other species and in light of extra concern about the well-being of nonhuman primates. It is appropriate to watch carefully neural studies that transplant human cells to primate brains, but the rationale for heightened oversight relates more to the well-being of the animal than to concerns about human dignity.

Chimeric research can touch core values, especially for those who do not accept embryo research in general or for those who draw a bright line between human and nonhuman species. To respect these values, it is essential to inform donors of gametes and embryos in advance if their donations might be used in combination with animal cells in chimera studies. To protect donor autonomy, donors must receive information about the nature and purpose of research, even if only broadly stated, in order to give informed consent for their gametes or embryos to be used in research (see, e.g., National Institutes of Health 1994; Ethics Committee 1997; Ethics Committee 2002). A recent examination of consent forms used by six institutions with ES cell lines listed on the NIH Registry, however, revealed that none informed donors that the cells derived from donated embryos might be used in human-nonhuman chimeric work (Streiffer 2008). A sample statement would let potential donors know that "human ESCs and/or cell lines might be used in research involving genetic manipulation of the cells or the mixing of human and nonhuman cells in animals models" (Streiffer 2008, 45).

At present no credible link exists between human-nonhuman chimeric research and the creation of an animal with human features. The consideration of regulatory policies or restrictions would more productively occur after evidence is available to inform the deliberations (Peters 2006). At present such speculation does not translate to a policy problem. The situation lacks imminence, credible focusing events, advocates, and a receptive national mood. Policy adjustments such as not allowing animal recipients of human ES cells to breed with one another may serve more to telegraph self-regulation by those closest to the science than to impose critically important restrictions.

In summary, proportionality is evident in the policy context for research on human-nonhuman chimeras. Deliberations about and oversight of chimeras are based more on evidence than are other types of early ISR, as seen in the following chapters. Some observers believe the research raises significant philosophical questions about what it is to be human (Baylis and Robert 2007, 44), but others are more skeptical (Greely et al. 2007). As one participant observed when called on to consult with the Committee on Guidelines on the matter of chimeras in ES-cell research, "My guess is that it will be a fairly minor point for your committee— something you need to discuss but not a major concern" (Board on Life Sciences and Board on Health Sciences Policy 2004, 1). This chapter does not belie this observation. At present, objections as well as justifications can be addressed through deliberation and minor adjustments to default policies if evidence indicates a persuasive need to do so.

Hybrids

THE *IDEA* OF A HYBRID is a powerful symbol, and the animal-human hybrid is a particularly well-known metaphor for research run amok. The thought of hybrids gives skeptics reasons to be wary about biotechnology; for example, in a 2004 report the President's Council on Bioethics (PCB) urged a "bright line" to be drawn against fertilizing human eggs with animal sperm or vice versa: "One bright line should be drawn at the creation of animal-human hybrid embryos, produced ex vivo by fertilization of human egg by animal (for example, chimpanzee) sperm (or the reverse)" (President's Council on Bioethics 2004, 220).

The animal-human hybrid is a sufficiently disconcerting scenario as to have been equated in the early years of modern biotechnology with the worst outcomes at the bottom of the slippery slope. The hybrid is a metaphor for biotechnology leading to the downgrading and depersonalization of humans as work horses or, conversely, to the elevation of animals to traits of greater cunning, prowess, and aggression. It is a symbol of uncertainty about the biotechnological future, and it has provoked calls by some to enact legally enforced bans to ensure that hybrids not be created.

The targeting of hybrids for regulatory limits is itself ironic given the chasm between actual and imagined hybrids. Technically, a hybrid is an organism resulting from fertilization of the egg of one species with the sperm of another. Under this definition, true hybrids are rare; they are not easy to create, and there is little need if any for them in biomedical research. The imagined hybrid, however, presents dramatic fodder for fiction and fantasy, especially as typified by the humanzee, which would in fact meet the criteria for a hybrid. Nevertheless, not even so-called hybrids in fiction meet these criteria. H. G. Wells's novel, *The Island of*

Dr. Moreau, for example, features the Leopard Man, Hairy Man, Swine Man, Swine Woman, Saint Bernard Dog Man, and others who represent hybrids. They are a fictional form of multispecies chimeras, however, not hybrids. Dr. Moreau created the beast people by subjecting animals to crude cut-and-paste surgery using tissue and organ transplantation, not by cross-fertilization (Wells 1993).

A satirical Internet image following the denunciation of animal-human hybrids in the 2006 U.S. Presidential address pitched Human-Animal Hybrid t-shirts featuring the cartoon profile of a monkey walking on all fours. Although the vertically curled tail and the four-legged gait were those of a monkey, the feet and necktie hanging from the creature's neck were detectably human (Tester 2006). Even this being was not necessarily a hybrid, however: It more likely reflected high-tech transgenic manipulations and low-tech sartorial choices rather than full fertilization using monkey and human gametes. In short, actual animal-human hybrids may be as scarce in fiction as they are in fact.

HYBRIDS IN NATURE

Hybrids are organisms in which a member of one species contributes the egg and a member of a second species contributes the spermatozoan. Hybrids have genes from each parental species in all their cells; the cells, in other words, "carry roughly equal genetic contributions from two distinct species" (ISSCR 2006, 14). Animal-animal hybrids are harder to produce than chimeras and will survive only if fertilization is between closely related species (ISSCR 2006, 14). Species are regarded as "groups of interbreeding natural populations that are reproductively isolated from other such groups" (Ridley 1996, 403). An array of biological and social barriers stands in the way of interspecies reproduction, including differing numbers of chromosomes and other hurdles that make successful hybridization between animal species rare. Intraspecies cross-bred animals, on the other hand, are relatively common, but they are not technically hybrids because their parents are different subspecies within the same species. A Great Dane, a Basset hound, and a Chihuahua, for example, are all subspecies of the domesticated dog, *Canis lupus familiaris* (Items of Interest n.d., 1).

Although hybrids rarely occur in nature, they can occur with the assistance of breeders. For example, in the 1800s, breeders in India interbred tigers and lions as gifts for English monarchs (Liger n.d., 1). Because such animals live in different parts of the world, they would not normally mate. Approximately a dozen ligers—the offspring of a male lion and female tiger (*Panthera X leogris*)—exist in the world today, including a half-ton feline reputed to be the "biggest cat in the world" (www.foundationTV. co.uk/brilliantcreatures/ser5/show4item3.html). The Indian government outlawed interspecies breeding of large cats in 1985 after pressure from wildlife protection groups (Tigon n.d., 2). Other *Panthera* hybrids include the jaglion, leotig, and liguar (*Panthera* Hybrid n.d.). A more well-known hybrid is the mule, which is the offspring of a male donkey and a female horse (a hinny is the offspring of a male horse and a female donkey). The horse and donkey share a genus (*Equus*), but they are from different species. Very rarely, the mating of a goat (genus *Ovis*) and sheep (genus *Capra*) has been reported to produce live offspring (Geep n.d.).

Artificial insemination and in vitro fertilization (IVF) are used to produce animal-animal hybrids if different mating cues and rituals prevent copulation. For example, the ARC Centre for Kangeroo Genomics in Australia uses IVF and intracytoplasmic sperm injection to breed hybrid kangaroos for purposes of genetic mapping (ARC Centre for Kangaroo Genomics n.d.). Breeders also use a method of transferring young kangaroos of one species to the pouches of kangaroos of a different species. The young then become accustomed to the substitute species and will mate with members of that species when older (ARC Centre for Kangaroo Genomics n.d.).

Even these and other methods cannot always overcome physiological characteristics of animals of different species, such as different numbers of chromosomes, which make some interspecies reproduction impossible. A species, after all, is defined in part by the ability of its members to reproduce and create fertile offspring (Mayr 1982, 273). Moreover, animal-animal hybrids rarely survive (Committee on Guidelines 2005, 32), and there is no scientific or medical urgency to create animal-animal hybrids. Instead, commercial interests motivate cross breeding, such as creating ligers or tigons for circus attractions and beefalo for new meat products. Other hybrid matings of hoofed animals include the zonkey (zebra/donkey), zebroid (zebra/horse), zetland (zebra/pony), yakow (cow/yak), and cama (camel/llama).

HYBRIDS IN RESEARCH

At present there appears to be no rationale for creating animal-human hybrids in research. Members of the group that produced the U.K. report on humans and chimeras "were of the opinion that there is no scientific case for true interspecies hybrids" (U.K. Department of Health 2007b, Appendix H 5.7–5.9). The Wellcome Trust conveyed the same message: "full sexual hybrids between human and animal gametes would not develop beyond early preimplantation stages. It is hard to see what scientific information would be gained from such an experiment" (United Kingdom. Parliament 2007a). If there were some reason to combine human and nonhuman biological properties, this would be done by other methods such as transgenics, not by hybridization. Nevertheless, perhaps in order to protect flexibility in research, the U.K. House of Commons defeated a proposed ban on the creation of human-nonhuman hybrids in 2008 (Henderson and Elliott 2008).

One tangential technique, which yields a so-called humster, has been practiced for nearly thirty years and has been shielded from regulations that bar the creation of animal-human hybrids in the United Kingdom and other countries. The "humster" assay or hamster oocyte penetration (HOP) test was first reported in 1982 by French fertility doctors who used hamster eggs to evaluate the ability of human male spermatozoa to penetrate eggs (Assay for Sperm Quality 2000, 3). The hamster eggs, with zona removed, are kept in culture. If the sperm penetrate, the resulting entity, a "humster," is a fertilized one-cell egg (zygote). This "cross-species system" is an alternative to using scarce human eggs in vitro. By convention the humster is destroyed before it divides into two cells.

Thinking about Dignity
To the extent that commentary on animal-human hybrids exists, it can be said to fall on one of two poles of the animal-human spectrum. At one pole is the microscopic near-hybrid, the humster. On the other is the thought of a human-nonhuman primate, generally called a humanzee,

lumbering about as an adult after birth. This is an exceedingly remote prospect both in the scientific sense and in lack of human motivation to create such a being.

The two poles of humanzee and humster are separated by significant and obvious differences. The humanzee is a fantasy with a spooky outcome that involves a species close to humans. The humster, on the other hand, is created by a minor technique with a prosaic outcome that involves a species distant from humans. Creation of the former would pose substantial ethical dilemmas; the latter poses no significant dilemmas. The former would meet the criteria for a hybrid, but the latter would be a hybrid in spirit rather than fact because the hamster egg and human spermatozoan would not combine, and, even if they did, the resulting organism, with two widely disparate species as donors, could not develop into a viable entity (National Institutes of Health 1994, 96).

Because regulations in various countries bar animal-human hybrid research, and because such policy generally lacks a narrative that spells out intent and justification, it may be helpful here to explore ethical challenges made to bar the creation of animal-human hybrids. One of these is the supposition that animal-human hybrids would intrude on human dignity. U.S. Senate Bill 1373, for example, would have barred the creation of a "hybrid human-animal embryo" on the grounds, among other things, that it would endanger "respect for human dignity and the integrity of the human species" (U.S. Senate 2005b).

To bridge the gap between factual humsters and fantasy-based humanzees, a middle category will be added here for the sake of discussion—research that pairs the gametes of humans and an intermediate species such as dogs. Although this is largely an academic exercise, it helps identify and explore the reasons behind policies. Would creating a human-hamster, human-canine, or human-chimpanzee embryo for research purposes violate human dignity? Although the term "embryo" is used, a more accurate term might be "embryonic entity," an early-stage organism with gametes from a human and a second species that has cleaved beyond two cells. "Entity" reflects uncertainty about whether the organism would be technically an embryo.

First, would creating a human-hamster embryonic entity violate human dignity, if dignity is defined as protecting capabilities that are part of humans' inherent worth (Nussbaum 2008, 357)? This entity would be created to meet a valid medical goal of humans—fertility assessment—which would in turn be part of the human interest in procreation. This seems to respect human interests. More importantly, this entity would not have the makings of a human, namely an intact human embryo, at its base. The humster assay brings together but does not integrate gametes from two distant species, which means no genetic mingling takes place. Even if mingling did take place, the entity could not develop into a viable organism. It would not be a real human, hamster, or humster. The human-hamster fertilized zygote is two steps removed from humans: (1) it is not a potentially viable entity, and (2) it is not even a human embryo. Thus, human dignity would not be violated any more than by other research or tests on human sperm. The procedure ends at the zygote stage, there are valid justifications for the test, and the species are distant. It involves gametes rather than intact human embryos. By convention and, in some cases, law, practitioners do not allow the entity to divide beyond two cells.

Would creating a human-canine embryonic entity for research purposes then violate human dignity? By the above reasoning it would not because the organism would not be a human embryo and might not even be a functioning hybrid embryo. It might continue dividing, but it would degrade. The human embryo is regarded in U.S. policy, for example, as a *"potential human being* worthy of special respect" (Ethics Advisory Board 1979; *Davis v. Davis* 1992). If the entity does not have the potential to become a human being, even if allowed to develop beyond the zygote stage, it would not be a human embryo.

Might hybrid embryos be considered less contentious than human embryos in research precisely because they are not fully human? In some ways the discussion of hybrids parallels proposals to use nonviable embryos in human ES-cell and therapeutic cloning studies. For example, embryos donated by couples at fertility clinics that are no longer viable but continue dividing could be one source (Holden and Vogel 2004, 2176). Another source is use of the technique of "altered nuclear transfer" to create an embryo that could produce ES cells but could not develop further because researchers would have knocked out a key developmental gene from the donor's nuclear DNA before the nucleus was transferred to the enucleated egg (Hall 2006). This technique would enable

ES cells to be retrieved, but it would prevent further development and implantation (ISSCR 2006, 13). Although some observers resist deliberately creating nonviable embryos (Melton, Daley, and Jennings 2004; Holden and Vogel 2004; President's Council on Bioethics 2005a), others see this as a promising way of securing ES cells while avoiding the destruction of human embryos. Animal-human hybrid embryonic entities are analogous if they are not viable and cannot develop to an organism. A nonviable status weakens the claim that using the entities would mar human dignity.

Some would counter that a nonviable embryo (because of an abnormality or an intervention that ended its ability to develop) is still an embryo. According to this point of view, it is no defense that the embryo cannot survive, and all protections should be given whether the embryo is viable or not (Parliament of the Commonwealth 2006a, 2006b). A more common view presumably is that if ES cells ethically can be retrieved from viable human embryos donated by couples in fertility clinics, they can certainly be retrieved from nonviable embryos as well. As to the main question, objections based on dignity do not persuasively make the case that the creation of a human-canine embryonic entity for research should be prohibited. This is not to say the act would be ethical or justifiable; it is simply to say claims of human dignity are not germane in the absence of a human embryo. Nor would creating a human-canine embryonic entity violate human dignity by misusing human gametes. Sperm and eggs contain only half the information needed for a full genome and are not in themselves integral to dignity, although the method of procuring gametes does matter.

Third, would creating a human-chimpanzee embryonic entity for research purposes violate human dignity? In this situation it is at least remotely possible that the entity could be capable of development and therefore be more akin to an embryo, but this cannot be tested. As the ISSCR noted, "hybrids are only likely to survive if the genetic contributions derive from closely related species . . . the greatest concern would be for experiments that entail creation of hybrids between humans and closely related nonhuman primates" (ISSCR 2006, 14). The entity here would not be a human embryo, but it might be an embryo. The key argument against this—that it might lead to the birth of a hybrid entity—is addressed below. For now, the question is whether the creation of this embryo for research and destruction would violate dignity.

Here again, dignity is not an especially effective concept with which to assess the ethics of this hypothetical research because one is not dealing with a human embryo. If embryo research is accepted in principle, then it is awkward to conclude that research on a "lesser" entity violates human dignity. But one is dealing with a potentially viable embryo from two highly developed species that share some capabilities. An analysis based on norms of embryo research may be a better guide. Does a strong or compelling reason exist for creating an entity rich with symbolic meaning for a research process for which consensus is lacking? Have less intrusive alternatives been exhausted? Do the rationale and likely benefit outweigh the interests of one species that is fully protected by legally mandated research regulations (humans) and by another that is accorded significant protections (chimpanzees)? Have the creators of such a hybrid embryo borne the burden of proof? These reasons for not going ahead with research are arguably more persuasive than a reason based on human dignity. Human and nonhuman donors should be protected, compelling reasons should exist to pursue the research, and alternative methods of addressing the scientific questions should be exhausted.

Thinking about Procreation

The fearsome image here is of transferring a human-animal hybrid embryo to a woman's uterus for potential procreation. The archetypal hybrid is the humanzee, as it has appeared in popular culture and in policy discussions. The being would be a humanzee (if the father is human) or chimphuman (if the mother is human). Or, given the gentler disposition of bonobos, it could be a humobo (with human father) or bonobuman (with human mother). This matter arose for consideration in 2003 when the PCB devoted a special session to chimeras. The council chair asked members at the beginning of the meeting about the morality of creating a humanzee (President's Council on Bioethics 2003b, 2). If creating a humanzee would be wrong, why would it be wrong?

Kass, the PCB chair at the time, and others have articulated a "repugnance argument" to suggest that certain acts in biotechnology are wrong if the idea of performing them elicits repugnance. To Kass, such an emotional reaction is a beacon of right and wrong, and in his well-known phrase, humans should recognize a certain "wisdom of repugnance" that guides moral action (Kass 1997). Certainly the idea of creating a humanzee, if such a thing were possible, would be shocking and offensive. But repugnance has weaknesses as a guide to what is moral or immoral (Karpowicz, Cohen, and van der Kooy 2005; Macklin 2006). Do reasons not grounded in repugnance exist as effective challenges to animal-human hybrids? One proffered here is that procreating human-nonhuman primates is wrong because it would bring significant harm to the hybrid and would offer no counterbalancing benefits.

To explain, the formation of a human-nonhuman primate hybrid would not happen in natural conditions. Even if a human had the yen to mate with a nonhuman primate, no infant would result from the liaison. Humans and chimpanzees do not procreate under natural conditions; a debate is ongoing about whether humans even interbred with the Neanderthals (*Homo neanderthalensis*), who were closer in appearance and genetic composition to today's humans (*Homo sapiens)* than chimpanzees and other nonhuman primates (Wade 2006, A10; Wilford 2006).

Natural reproduction between human and chimpanzee does not occur for social and biological reasons. Species are defined partly by their reproductive isolation. Normally, different species do not interbreed even if they live in the same region (Ridley 1996, 403). Reproductive isolation comes from characteristics that foreclose interspecies attraction, such as different mating seasons, lack of sexual attraction, and gametes from one species that are not viable in the sexual tract of another species. If intercourse does occur between two nonhuman species, hybrid zygotes are unlikely to survive; even if a birth were to occur between two animal species, the offspring would likely not have functional gametes and would be sterile. Chimpanzees and humans have different numbers of chromosomes (forty-six for humans and forty-eight for chimpanzees), which is a significant barrier to conception (Silver 2006). Still, Richard Dawkins suggests that producing such a hybrid "cannot be ruled out as impossible" (Dawkins 2009).

In vitro fertilization and other interventions could possibly overcome social barriers to hybrid mating, but they would leave unresolved the biological matters of zygote viability and the embryo's ability to implant. The matter of incentives is also apropos. Medical professionals would need expertise, equipment, and motivation to undertake an activity that would defy social conventions and that would be extremely risky. Remarkable time and perseverance would be needed to bring about a humanzee, and any motivation to do this is mystifying. As noted by the Committee on Guidelines, "no one proposes to generate interspecies hybrids involving human gametes, even if it were possible" (Committee on Guidelines 2005, 32).

Undeniably, an animal-human hybrid would be unsettling, with a truly unpredictable outcome. It would be more unsettling than cloning, parthenogenesis, or genetic alterations where the outcomes would be relatively more predictable if safety were assured and extensive animal research were undertaken beforehand. In fact cloning is condemned precisely because it might be too predictable for the offspring and deprive him or her of the "right to an open future." But an animal-human hybrid would be unpredictable in that it would reflect a fifty-fifty genetic split. One could not predict which genes the offspring would inherit from the chimpanzee and which from the human. People who use science fiction to visualize a humanzee tend to think he or she would inherit aggressiveness and musculature from the chimpanzee. But fertilization means chimpanzee and human genomes are united in each body cell. This is not targeted DNA splicing, in which genes for aggression, musculature, or other traits could theoretically be introduced in a more controlled manner.

The offspring born from chimp and human parents could inherit any mixture of genes from each parent, just as human offspring regularly do. In human procreation, one cannot predict whether a child will inherit the musical ability of the mother or the deep voice of the father. The same would apply for a humanzee. Assuming a humanzee would be more human-like than chimp-like, one could not predict whether the child would huf-huf to communicate like the chimpanzee or inherit a more modulated speaking voice from the human parent. Would the child's arms be longer, like the calf-length arms of the chimpanzee parent, or shorter, like the arms of the human parent? Would the child engage in lip smacking or the lip flip characteristic of chimpanzees when excited? (Gelada Baboon 2006).

Traits depend on which genes are dominant, how the genes interrelate, their pattern of expression, and how they interact with environmental influences. Also, the effects of imprinting are uncertain. Here genes may or may not be expressed, depending on which parent provided the dominant gene. Just as the paternal/maternal parentage for animal hybrids affects the outcome (e.g., the tigon with a tiger father and lion mother and the liger with a lion father and a tiger mother), so might the outcome differ depending on whether the chimp gamete was from a male (chimphuman) or from a female (humanzee) (Humanzee n.d., 1).

Studies of hybrid primates do not portend well for a chimp-human mixture. For example, investigators who studied the offspring of interbreeding in the wild between gelada monkeys (*Theropithecus gelada*) and hamadryas baboons (*Papio hamadryas*) found that the offspring were "large but developmentally normal" and fell midway between the two parent species in "skull and tooth form and to a lesser extent in postcranial proportions" (Jolly et al. 1997). Although the offspring were apparently healthy, they had a hybrid appearance, which would not augur well for the offspring of a chimpanzee and human. A study of seventeen hybrid offspring between *Papio* and *Macaca* genera and *Theropithecus* genera showed mixed features of all offspring (Markarjan, Isakov, and Kondakov 1974). As described by the investigators: "Hybrids between the *Papio* and *Macaca* genera resembled baboons according to the body build and colour of eyes, but according to the form of head, face, hair colour, sexual skin and ischial callosities they resembled macaques." The offspring of *Papio* and *Theropithecus* were fertile, but those between *Macaca* and *Papio* were not.

The results of a human-nonhuman primate fertilization, in short, would harm the offspring. A child who is more human-like than chimplike would have visible physical features of two species and presumably would have mixed internal physiological features and cognitive abilities as well. A child who is more chimp-like than human-like would be subject to mores for treating nonhuman primates. In either case, combining the gametes of both species would violate the core bioethical principle of nonmaleficence because it would bring both physiological and psychological harms. No imaginable benefit would accrue except existence, and even that would be hard to justify.

Thinking about Species

What would be the impact of human-animal hybridization on animals? Looking at animal-animal hybrids gives clues about the unpredictability and fundamental changes that come from hybridization. For example, tigers and lions do not share the same territory, so they ordinarily do not mate. If assisted by breeders, however, the fertilization of lion sperm and tiger eggs could lead to a liger. A liger is very large, with male ligers weighing up to 1000 pounds. This contrasts to the average 400 pounds for male lions.

One explanation for the growth dysplasia is that imprinting affects which genes are expressed depending on the parent from whom they were inherited (Liger n.d.; Liger.org 2009). An explanation based on evolutionary theory supposes that lions live in prides and female lions mate with more than one male so their cubs have different fathers. Male lions benefit if their genes survive, so they have an advantage if their offspring are large; consequently, their genes promote growth. Female lions benefit by having most of their cubs survive. Therefore, the female's genes inhibit growth so more cubs will survive gestation. Tigers, on the other hand, are solitary, and the females mate with only one male. As a result, there will be just one cub. The males do not compete with other males, so their genes do not need to promote growth, and the female does not need to inhibit the growth of the developing cub (Liger n.d.; Liger.org 2009).

With a liger, the genetic balance unravels. If a male lion mates with a female tiger, his genes will program large growth but the female tiger's genes will not inhibit the growth. Therefore, the offspring will eventually be larger than the parents. If a male tiger and a female lion (tigon) mate, his genes do not promote growth, and her genes inhibit growth. This may affect physical well-being. The resulting offspring will be smaller than the parents and may be "less robust" as well (Liger n.d.; Liger.org 2009). In addition, the welfare of the tiger that gestates and gives birth to the large liger is surely part of the evaluation.

Hybridization may also affect the psychic well-being of ligers, although this can only be inferred. For example, tigers like to swim but lions do not (Liger n.d.; Liger.org 2009). What would be the swimming preferences of hybrid offspring? The communication abilities of the animals may be affected, inasmuch as "tigers 'cuff,' lions roar" (1). Diana Schaub wonders whether the animals are affected by "conflicting instincts, mixed vocabularies, and incompatible behaviors and ways of life" (Schaub 2006, 35). Some observers speculate that ligers may have behavioral problems, such as confusion and depression from inheriting the social nature of the lion and the solitary nature of the tiger. Schaub considers the hybrid's stake in life: "Lions are social; tigers are solitary. What is a liger or tigon to do?" (Schaub 2006, 35). Until ethologists develop more refined methods of measuring animal well-being, answers about the impact of hybridization remain incomplete.

A more common hybrid, the mule, has a reputation for being ornery, but mules have no outward signs of deformities or physical problems. The jury is out on the effect of hybridization on the mule's temperament. Defenders of mules say they are good-natured and have received wrongful personality reviews. If indeed they are ornery, says Schaub, "Maybe mules are mulish for good reason. Maybe they aren't happy about their betwixt and between lot in life" (President's Council on Bioethics 2005c; Schaub 2006, 35).

Many bison in the United States have cattle genes resulting from crossbreeding by ranchers who wanted their cows to inherit genes that make bison resistant to some diseases and parasites (Robbins 2007). Most of the approximately three hundred thousand bison now in the United States have cattle genes. Even though the genes make up only 1 percent of bison genes, this could harm bison by making them less resistant, and it could affect both their weight and fertility. The genetic makeup of the bison cannot be predicted because "their immunological response can be all over the place" (Robbins 2007). One geneticist was quoted as saying "When you mix up two different genomes, you get a lot of different traits, and it's not completely predictable" (Robbins 2007). Hybrid vigor can lead to a more robust animal, but this does not happen when cattle and bison are cross-bred. Thus, hybridization would have impacts on animals, but the nature of these impacts is not necessarily predictable. This means animal interests should be part of the calculation if ever one assesses a need for human-nonhuman hybrid research.

Policy Directions

The PCB, after calling for a bright line at animal-human hybrids, recommended that the U.S. Congress "prohibit the production of a hybrid human-animal embryo by fertilization of human egg by animal sperm or of animal egg by human sperm" (President's Council on Bioethics 2004, 221). Members of the U.S. Senate introduced Senate Bill 659 and Senate Bill 1373 in 2005 to make it a crime to create a human chimera. The bills included two meanings of chimeras (of eight total) that were actually hybrids: (1) "a hybrid human-animal embryo produced by fertilizing a human egg with non-human sperm" and (2) "a hybrid human-animal embryo produced by fertilizing a non-human egg with human sperm."

Concerns about animal-human hybrids have been expressed for years, and hybrids are prohibited by law in Australia, Germany, France, and Italy, among other countries (ISSCR 2006; U.K. Department of Health 2007b, Appendix C). Some laws forbid the creation of a hybrid embryo for research purposes, whereas others forbid only the transfer of the embryo to a uterus for procreation. Australia's Prohibition of Human Cloning for Reproduction and the Regulation of Human Embryo Research Amendment Act 2006 forbids creating a human-nonhuman chimeric embryo without a license, but the only license that can be granted is for fertility assessment (humster test) as long as the entity does not develop to the first mitotic division (Hinxton Group 2008).

Canada's law on assisted reproductive technologies and research prohibits the creation of a hybrid embryo for the purpose of reproduction or the transfer of one to a human or nonhuman uterus (Canada/ Government 2004). The law defines a hybrid as a human egg fertilized by a nonhuman spermatozoon or vice versa. Some nations, including the United States, are silent on the matter, as are most advisory groups. The HFE Act 1990 of the United Kingdom allowed the mixing of human and nonhuman gametes only "in pursuance of a licence" (Human Genetics Advisory Committee 1998, 34). In the process of revising the HFE Act in May 2008, the U.K. House of Commons defeated an amendment to a bill that would have banned the creation of human-nonhuman hybrid embryos (Henderson and Elliott 2008).

Humsters have accompanied hybrid regulations in the United Kingdom as a footnote or comment with an asterisk, starting in 1984 when the Warnock Commission carved an exception for the humster test by recommending that "trans-species fertilization" could be licensed if used to alleviate infertility or subfertility, as long as the "development of any hybrid [is] terminated at the two cell stage" (Warnock 1985, 81). The HFE Act 1990 adopted this principle by allowing the test in facilities licensed to perform it provided that "the result of the mixed gametes is destroyed when the test is complete (and definitely no later than the two cell stage)" (U.K. Department of Health 2006, 24). The HFE Act 2008 allows mixing of human and animal eggs or sperm as long as the resulting entity is not allowed to develop beyond fourteen days or be transferred to a human or animal uterus (U.K. HFE Act 2008 [Part 1.4(2)(3)(3)]; Vogel 2008).

In the United States the Human Embryo Research Panel (HERP) in 1994 regarded tests using hamster eggs or the eggs of other animals to test sperm penetrability as ethically acceptable as long as the organism did not develop beyond the one-cell stage (National Institutes of Health 1994, 96). Another potential test is to study sperm chromosomes by injecting human spermatozoa into mouse preembryos at the two-cell stage. This does not fit the definition of hybrid used here. Investigators presumably would use transgenetic modifications rather than hybridization to mix human and animal DNA.

Advance prohibitions on hybrids are a form of prior restraint. To make research procedures criminal in the absence of persuasive evidence about imminence and serious benefit-harm calculations is serious in biomedical research. A legislative review committee in Australia, for example, noted that the matter of animal-human hybrids was prohibited but had only been mentioned in a "few of the submissions and hearings" (Legislation Review Committee 2005, 154). Nevertheless, "there was an implicit understanding that the creation of such entities could be of concern to the community," so the committee recommended that the creation of hybrid embryos for reproduction "continue to be prohibited." It did include an exception for the hamster or its equivalent by allowing an animal egg to be fertilized under license to the first mitotic division with human sperm in order to test sperm quality. This decision typifies a key question: When is it an appropriate time to begin thinking about and crafting policy relating to possible but not foreseeable research and development?

The wisdom of advance prohibitions is open to debate. On one hand, advance bans draw a firm line against applications thought to be morally untenable, which can be compelling. On the other hand, advance prohibitions are generally not open to nuances, and they hobble lines of inquiry if researchers reach more widely than necessary to avoid violating the law. They cannot easily be changed and are hard to interpret in light of changing technologies. Proportionality is not evident in the policy context for animal-human hybrids. The science is speculative, and focusing events have not signaled the need to move the issue to the policy agenda. Although anticipatory bans can telegraph clear lines and can address moral concerns, they may convey undeserved distrust about the motives of researchers in biotechnology.

SUMMARY

Although the term "hybrid" brings to mind fanciful creatures, the reality is far less sensational. A hybrid—referring strictly to the combination of eggs and sperm from two different species—is difficult to produce and to keep alive. Moreover, a great gap exists between what is feared and what is real. The humanzee and the humster represent two opposing ends of the debate spectrum, and the two are so dramatically different that they almost merit separate categories. The humanzee embodies the type of adult, aggressive creature in the popular culture that comes to mind with the thought of hybrids. Yet such a creature has never been seriously considered, and no justification exists for cobbling one together through fertilization. The humster, on the other hand, proves useful in medical settings and is not objectionable.

This chapter concludes that human-nonhuman hybrids do not present a genuine policy issue. Missing are focusing events based on scientific studies, a community of advocates, and a national mood demanding protection from hybrids. Despite recent calls in the United States to ban animal-human hybrids, the topic has not changed over time, and no newsworthy events reflect scientific developments. As contrasted with chimeras, the scales are out of balance, with broad prohibitions in some countries on one hand and no signs of imminence or motives for creating ethically problematic hybrids on the other.

Hybrids are perhaps more interesting as a symbol rather than as a potential scientific development. Studies exploring the metaphorical power of hybrids and reasons for visceral reactions to them would be welcome for their insight into attitudes toward biotechnology, the nature of species, and why early ISR provokes concerns. If the hybrid is a symbol of angst about interspecies beings, exploring various meanings of an "animal-human hybrid" would infuse new material to existing debates.

Cybrids, Cross-Species Embryo Transfer, and Transgenics

WHILE RESEARCHING HIS DAUGHTER'S MYSTERIOUS disease that brought with it seizures and kidney breakdown, James Reston Jr. noticed this headline in the *New York Times*: "Human-Cow Hybrid Cells Are Topic of Ethics Panel" (Reston 2006, 183). Looking for answers for his daughter, Reston responded with bafflement: "To this nonscientist, it seemed as if medical science was on the road to producing Minotaurs in the new millennium." At issue was something more prosaic, but the headline highlighted the sensation that comes with novel interspecies prospects. This chapter looks at three topics that are part of policy deliberations but have not captured either the strong academic interest in chimeras or the distortions in the public imagination about hybrids. For organizational purposes, these three topics are grouped into a single chapter: creation of cybrids, cross-species transfer of embryos, and transgenics.

CYBRIDS

The article spotted by Reston on human-cow hybrid cells referred to the experimental use of animal eggs to study somatic cell nuclear transfer (SCNT) (cloning) techniques as a method for procuring ES cells. In this technique, somatic cell nuclei are transferred to enucleated eggs, and the eggs are activated via an electric or chemical charge. The entity begins cleaving, and when it reaches a certain stage, the cells aggregate to an inner cell mass that, for a short period of time, contains undifferentiated ES cells. The eventual clinical goal is to coax the derived cells to differentiate to whatever specialized cells the patient needs and then to transfer them to him or her. Because the cells originated from the patient, they will share the same genome and be compatible, which will free the patient from requiring immunosuppressive drugs.

More basic research is needed before many clinical trials stemming from this technique can commence. A significant hurdle for this research is the difficulty of obtaining human eggs. Might animal eggs be a substitute? If so, they could be used to create entities from which ES cells might be derived. Variously called a "pseudohybrid," "interspecies embryo," "cytoplasmic hybrid embryo," "cybrid," "interspecies cytoplasmic hybrid," and "nuclear-cytoplasmic hybrid," a term used informally in the United Kingdom will be adopted here: cybrid (U.K. House of Commons 2007, 6, 20). Cybrids are "embryos created by removing the nucleus of an animal egg and inserting the nucleus of an adult cell from a different individual (and possibly of a different species)" (U.K. Department of Health 2007b, glossary).

The process of creating cybrids is informally called "interspecies SCNT" or iSCNT (Vogel 2006, 155). Using readily accessible animal eggs could speed studies geared to other ends as well, such as understanding the mechanisms behind diseases linked to defects in mitochondrial DNA (mtDNA) or developing methods for reprogramming gene expression (U.K. Department of Health 2007b, Appendix H. 3.5).

Human eggs are generally in short supply for research. Although women may be motivated by feelings of altruism to donate eggs to couples trying to conceive, incentives to donate for research are less attractive, especially with compensation in doubt. Another source of eggs—those donated by women as part of their fertility care when they produce more eggs than they want to have fertilized—may not be sufficient because of poor quality that contributed to infertility in the first place (United Kingdom. Parliament 2007d).

Although hyperstimulation and other aspects of the process are for the most part safe, they pose short- and long-term risks for human donors that may not be outweighed by benefits if only a small number of eggs are retrieved (Spar 2007, 1290; United Kingdom. Parliament 2007e). This is particularly the case in light of the large number of eggs needed to proceed systematically with the research.

Some policy advisory groups have recommended against compensating egg donors beyond reimbursement for expenses (Spar 2007, 1290).

They are concerned that undue inducements could undercut the voluntary nature of the donation. In South Korea where researchers claimed—fraudulently it turned out—to have derived human ES cells from embryos created through SCNT, some of the egg donors were students of the lead investigator and may have experienced inappropriate pressures to donate. Concerns are also expressed about undue inducement for women with low incomes and for those enrolled in colleges and universities.

Policies at the California Institute for Regenerative Medicine originally forbade either cash or in-kind payment to women donating for ES-cell research, directing the ES-cell research oversight committee to confirm that "the donation of oocytes for research is done without valuable consideration either directly or indirectly" (California Institute for Regenerative Medicine 2007, sec. 1000095(b)[3]). The NAS cautioned against cash or in-kind payment, but it did allow reimbursement for expenses (Committee on Guidelines 2005, 110). Its reasons for restricting compensation were to promote public confidence in the process, acknowledge the risks of donation, and ensure consistency with practices in countries outside the United States and with California's funded stem cell research program (72). Other states also forbid payment to donors for SCNT research (Spar 2007, 1290; Lomax and Stayn 2008, 698).

Other observers and groups believe reasonable compensation is appropriate in light of the risks and inconvenience of egg donation, provided careful informed consent procedures are followed about physical and psychological risks (Robertson 2006). If donors can be compensated for fertility donation, writes one observer, it is an "absurd inconsistency" to deny compensation to those who donate for research (Spar 2007, 1291). The International Society for Stem Cell Research (ISSCR) regards payment as acceptable if the procedures are reviewed by the research oversight committee. One provision stipulates that recruitment must be monitored to "ensure that no vulnerable populations, for example, economically disadvantaged women, are disproportionately encouraged to participate as oocyte providers for research" (ISSCR 2006, section 11.5.b). To ensure that financial arrangements do not amount to undue inducement, "rigorous review" is necessary.

If resistance to compensation stays the same or spreads, the scarcity of human eggs for research will remain. With this scarcity in view, the

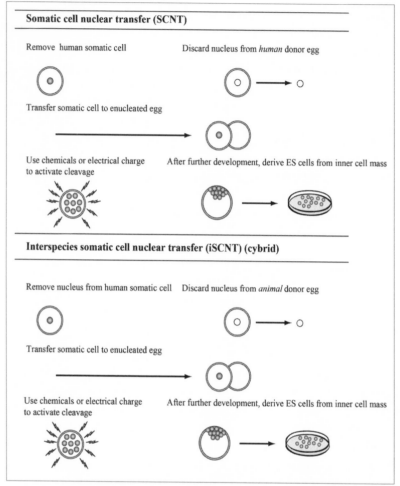

Figure 3.1.   **Obtaining Human ES Cells through SCNT and iSCNT (cybrid).**

use of animal eggs is an inexpensive and easily available alternative for research on therapeutic SCNT (see figure 3.1). Where an IVF clinic would "struggle to collect" ten to twenty donated eggs in a week, "hundreds of cow oocytes can be obtained from a single slaughterhouse every day" (United Kingdom. Parliament 2007g). If therapeutic SCNT proves to be effective and safe in preclinical investigation, the inquiry could progress to clinical trials and, eventually, to therapy. Without refinements in techniques, demand for human eggs may well escalate in these later stages of product development (Baylis 2008).

One estimate is that over thirty eggs would be needed to produce a cell line for each person being treated (U.K. House of Commons 2007, 30). Another is that, at least in the early research where the procedure is inefficient, "hundreds or even thousands of eggs" would be needed to create cell lines for small numbers of patients (United Kingdom. Parliament 2007d). To the extent that animal eggs can be used in early research, it has been proposed that a triage system be followed in which animal eggs are used now for exploratory studies and human eggs are saved for when they are really needed, such as in clinical trials (United Kingdom. Parliament 2007g).

Investigators have studied iSCNT between nonhuman species and have transferred nuclei from sheep, pigs, monkeys, rats, buffalo, and mice to enucleated cow eggs and have transferred nuclei from monkeys, cats, and chickens to enucleated rabbit eggs (Board on Life Sciences and Board on Health Sciences Policy 2004). Most of these studies resulted in blastocysts. For example, in transferring mouse cell nuclei to cow eggs, researchers in South Korea produced three blastocysts and one ES-cell line (Vogel 2006, 155). Researchers in the United Kingdom reported the following interspecies (nonhuman) cybrids that have developed to the blastocyst stage: "horse donor cell and cow oocyte, monkey donor cell and rabbit oocyte, various mammalian species and cow oocyte, mountain bongo antelope donor cell and cow oocyte, buffalo donor cell and cow oocyte, dog donor cell and yak or cow oocyte" (U.K. Department of Health 2007b, Appendix B. 1.2.4).

Less has been published regarding human somatic cells and animal eggs. In 2003 Chinese researchers reported combining nuclei from human skin cells and rabbit eggs to develop one hundred embryos and several stem-cell lines that had not yet been tested for stability and the capacity for "indefinite growth" (U.K. House of Commons 2007, 31; Committee on Guidelines 2005, 31). Selecting the best species for cybrids will depend on accessibility and compatibility with human development. Rabbit embryos, for example, have a developmental pace similar to that of humans (United Kingdom. Parliament 2007f).

It is possible that substitute methods of securing eggs will be available in the future, such as in vitro maturation of eggs from ovaries or from "egg-like" entities generated from ES cells. As Anne McLaren recounted, researchers have already derived eggs and sperm from mouse ES cells, which makes it conceivable the same could be done to generate human egg-like gametes (McLaren 2007). If these gametes are found to be safe and functional, they could help address the egg shortage for fertility research.

Another technique is to reprogram differentiated cells to produce what have been called induced pluripotent stem (iPS) cells. Using mice, investigators have changed a limited number of gene factors in mouse skin cells in order to reprogram the cells and induce the formation of pluripotent stem cells (Cyranoski 2007). These cells, like ES cells, are versatile. They can proliferate indefinitely in culture and develop into cells of the three germ layers (National Institutes of Health 2009). Investigators have also produced iPS cells using human somatic cells (Takahashi et al. 2007; Yu et al. 2007). Further studies are under way to identify and reduce risks associated with the procedures in order to set the stage for eventual clinical studies (Baker 2000; Hayden and Baker 2009). If somatic cells can be dedifferentiated to produce cells that are nearly like ES cells, this would obviate the need for eggs or embryos in producing cells and tissues for therapy that are compatible with the genome of the intended patient, who has provided the body cells.

Thinking about Dignity

In what ways, if any, might the creation of cybrids for research violate human dignity? Presumably, those who accord the embryo the same protections as a person and who regard the cybrid as an embryo would see this research as immoral and a violation of dignity, when defined as a violation of the person's right not to be treated as another's end. A representative of the Scottish Council on Human Bioethics (SCHB), an advisory group opposed to early interspecies research (ISR), asserted that animal-human embryo combinations are "not just a pile of cells," but instead have a "special moral status as a human person" and ought to be protected by the Council of Europe Convention on Human Rights and Biomedicine, which stipulates that embryos cannot be created and destroyed for research purposes (United Kingdom. Parliament 2007c).

Although the United Kingdom has not ratified the convention, the document holds particular import for those who object to research using human embryos.

The SCHB also referred to human dignity in particular, stating that animal-human combinations "could seriously undermine the whole concept of human dignity as defined by the United Nations Universal Declaration of Human Rights (United Kingdom. Parliament 2007c). The Preamble of the Declaration presumes the "inherent dignity" of all humans as the "foundation of freedom, justice and peace in the world." According to the SCHB, creating cybrids would be "crossing the species barrier" and would confuse the "general understanding of what it means to be a human person." Under this reasoning "human beings are generally considered to have a specific human dignity which nonhuman animals do not have." To mix human and nonhuman biological material at this early stage may "begin to undermine the whole distinction between human and nonhuman animals for which a different understanding of dignity exists" (United Kingdom. Parliament 2007c). Similarly, the Christian Action Research and Education organization in the United Kingdom has argued against cybrids because the blurring of human-nonhuman boundaries in research would "demean what is fully human by degrading the life in question with animal content" (United Kingdom. Parliament 2007h).

The Christian Medical Fellowship based its conclusion that using animal eggs would be immoral on religious grounds (United Kingdom. Parliament 2007i). Referring to the biblical concept of "according to their kinds," the Fellowship writes that "humans are the only animals made 'in the image of God,'" so a higher ethical standard is needed for them. The revulsion some people feel about human-nonhuman combinations applies to entities destroyed in laboratories as well as to those transferred for procreation: "a chimera of this type violates the natural order and should be prohibited, whether in vitro or in vivo" (United Kingdom. Parliament 2007i).

One response to dignity-based objections to cybrids is that the research would benefit humans by promoting the study of embryonic development, stem-cell functioning, interactions between the nucleus and cytoplasm, and the role of cytoplasm in cell reprogramming (United Kingdom.

Parliament 2007e). In addition some research now could obviate the need for cybrids in the future by educating investigators on how to remove animal cytoplasm and replace it with human cytoplasm from the cell that provided the nucleus, which would eliminate the nonhuman contribution (United Kingdom. Parliament 2007b). Another line of research is to learn how to dedifferentiate specialized cells to produce ES cells (what is now called iPS research) without having to use an egg to produce an embryo first (United Kingdom. Parliament 2007g). Thus the intention is to minimize the number of embryos used, reflecting a higher status for human embryos than for other cells.

A second response is that the cybrid's status as an embryo is contestable. If the cybrid is not a human embryo, human dignity would seemingly not be jeopardized. When President Clinton asked the NBAC in 1997 whether the human-cow embryo would be a human embryo, the commission concluded it did not have enough information to answer that question. In the United Kingdom, whether such an entity is a human embryo has direct policy implications. If it is an embryo, it would be brought into the relatively permissive regulatory structure of the HFE Act. If it is not an embryo, research on it could be forbidden altogether. To determine whether an entity is an embryo, the approach in the United Kingdom has been to look at the embryo itself rather than the technique used to generate it. As the HFE Act was written, "it is the nature of the embryo, and not the process by which it is created, that is critical to the question of whether it falls within the scope of the Act" (U.K. House of Commons 2007, 38). The House of Lords also stated that the HFE Act has jurisdiction over embryos created outside the body "regardless of how the embryos were created" (37).

The HFE Act has asserted that an embryo with a full human genome should be treated as a live human embryo "unless it could be clearly proved that the embryo could never be viable" (38). The HFE Act and Parliament have determined that the cybrid is a human embryo for purposes of the HFE Act because it has a full human genome and because the nonhuman mitochondrial contribution would fade early in embryonic development (39). Even if the cybrid is an embryo for policy purposes, it is not known whether it would be a viable embryo, where viability refers to the "normal potential to develop" of a transferred embryo (40).

British experts did not agree on whether a cybrid would be viable, saying it is "impossible to prove categorically" because it would be unethical and illegal in the United Kingdom to transfer the embryo to a woman's uterus (40). Still, cloning studies indicate that embryos resulting from nuclear transfer are "typically abnormal and often die during development" even if they yield apparently normal inner cell masses. If embryos created through SCNT with human nuclei and human eggs are "rarely... capable of developing to term," the same logically would hold true for human nuclei and nonhuman eggs, which is to say they would not be viable (ISSCR 2006, 13).

The objection that the mere presence of animal components would render cybrids a violation of human dignity is largely religious based and is not necessarily shared by all religions or by those who do not follow a religion (see, e.g., Cobbe 2007; Modell 2007). It also reflects a particular and contestable view of evolution that draws a clear line between humans and all other species (Dawkins 2009). A more inclusive ground for evaluating cybrid research would be to examine the intent, need, risks, and other elements of the research. A well-crafted investigation using a small number of embryos with an animal component for highly promising research would, in this calculation, be more ethically acceptable than a study on human embryos done for frivolous reasons with little regard for the number of embryos used and without an animal component.

Thinking about Procreation

Would the creation of cybrids for research be a step toward eventual use of cybrids for human procreation? Although not expressed as prevalently as for other forms of early ISR, this concern is evidenced by laws that forbid the transfer of a cybrid to the uterus of a woman or a female animal. The likelihood of anyone attempting to use a human-animal cybrid for reproduction is exceedingly remote, however, and its attendant risks would make this a peculiar choice. There is no insurmountable human egg shortage for fertility treatment, so there is no rationale to use animal eggs. Moreover, the safety could not be assured. If animal mitochondria remained, it is likely there would "be too much cell loss to maintain integrity of the embryo (assuming anyone was foolish enough to try to implant them)" (United Kingdom. Parliament 2007f).

The creation of cybrids melds with another ethically problematic matter, reproductive cloning, to which there is widespread resistance. In cloning, a somatic cell from a potential parent would be injected into an enucleated donor egg, activated, and transferred to the uterus of the would-be mother. As Jonathan Moreno put it, human cloning is "something every reputable scientist, science advocate, and science organization in the world is on record opposing" (Moreno 2006). Both legally based and voluntary lines have been drawn against cloning, and these lines are unlikely to be broken with human eggs, let alone with nonhuman eggs. If reproductive SCNT is ever deemed ethically acceptable, there would be no reason to use animal eggs when human eggs would be a safer and more acceptable alternative.

For these and other reasons, procreative use is not a probable outcome of cybrid research and is therefore not in itself a sufficient reason to bar the use of cybrids in research. As one ES-cell researcher put it, "These experiments don't make animals, they make cells" (quoted in Elias 2006). As another stated, "It's not our intention to create any bizarre cow-human hybrid; we want to use those cells to understand how to make human stem cells better" (BBC News 2007).

Thinking about Species

As noted above, an objection to cybrids is that they will lead to a "blurring of the important differences between what makes human and nonhuman life" (United Kingdom. Parliament 2007c). According to this objection the mere fact of nonhuman-human combinations in early ISR is determinative. No matter how minute the animal contribution in cybrid creation (e.g., 99.9 percent human and 0.1 percent nonhuman), the mere fact of a combination is significant, not the size of the fraction (Henderson and Elliott 2008).

A contrary view is that the human-nonhuman ratio matters. According to this view, creating cybrids is a relatively benign form of IRS that involves a less complex mingling of cells than do chimeras (where cells exist side by side) or hybrids (where nuclear DNA is mixed between species). According to McLaren, the eggs used to create cybrids are little more than "carriers of human nuclei" (McLaren 2007). A cybrid would have a "full human genome," and all cells would have the same human genes (United

Kingdom. Parliament 2007b). The animal cytoplasm would contribute only mtDNA, which has a separate genome and is the source of the cell's energy.

The exact interplay of the human and nonhuman material is open to question. Some scientists believe the presence of nonhuman mtDNA would have a significant impact in light of the vital biochemical role mtDNA plays in development and the fact that defects in mtDNA lead to serious illnesses. They surmise that the entities would not be "basically human" with a "few additional animal cells" (United Kingdom. Parliament 2007f). However, others surmise that animal mtDNA would "[make] very little contribution to the actual information content of the final cell" (U.K. House of Commons 2007, 39). Moreover because some human mtDNA would be attached to the human nucleus, the egg would have mitochondria from two species. As a result the nonhuman mitochondria would likely fade away, depending on the species and whether investigators tried to add to or reduce their presence (United Kingdom. Parliament 2007f). Potentially the "resulting embryo will eventually derive all of the gene products needed for development from the human genome" (United Kingdom. Parliament 2007g). In short the actual degree of blurring between species in the creation of cybrids is open to question. For critics of the research, this is beside the point. For supporters of the research, it renders minimal to nonexistent any ethical issues associated with the investigations.

Would the creation of cybrids have a harmful effect on animals? The impact on animal egg donors would not go beyond other uses of animals if investigators obtained eggs from places where pigs or other animals were destroyed for consumption or another purpose (Braga et al. 2007). More importantly, a ready source of eggs could facilitate ES-cell research and reduce the need for animals. For example, a ready source of eggs for procuring stem cells would enable drug toxicity testing on human cell lines rather than on animals, thereby reducing the numbers of animals needed for the tests. In addition cells derived from the iSCNT process also "should reduce the need for research on live animals as models for certain diseases" (U.K. House of Commons 2007, 29). If somatic cell nuclei from patients with Type 1 diabetes were transferred to enucleated cow eggs, the resulting stem cells derived from the blastocyst could be used to create

ES-cell lines specific to that disease for investigation (United Kingdom. Parliament 2007g).

Policy Directions

In the United States creating human-nonhuman cybrids is not illegal, but neither it nor SCNT using human eggs is funded by the federal government. The extent to which it is practiced by privately funded researchers is hard to assess because there is no disclosure requirement as there would be for publicly funded research.

In Massachusetts, Advanced Cell Technology patented a technique for transferring human nuclei to cow eggs (Robert 2006, 841). In 1997 when the NBAC studied cybrids from cow eggs, it concluded the procedure was unsafe and should not be done "at this time." Government personnel asked the NBAC chair to delete "at this time" from the report, which he declined to do. The phrase was deleted anyway, without the assent of the commissioners or its chair, in the final report to the president (Center for American Progress 2006, 13). This indicates intemperance toward the technique, at least from that presidential administration. The NAS concluded that if nonhuman eggs were used, the same norms and limits should be applied as for other ES-cell research, such as not allowing the entity to develop for more than fourteen days (Committee on Guidelines 2005, 35). In effect this equates the cybrid with an embryo.

Additionally as discussed in chapter 1, the regulatory scheme of the Food and Drug Administration (FDA) regards embryos that have been "more than minimally manipulated" as biological products. Further, these products have been "highly processed, [and] are used for other than their normal function" (Halme and Kessler 2006, 1730). In an untested assertion of its authority, the FDA has indicated it will not allow reproductive cloning to proceed (www.fda.gov/cber/ltr/aaclone.pdf). It has also placed a clinical hold on the transfer of ooplasm from a younger woman's egg to an older woman's egg to rejuvenate the egg and increase the odds of fertilization. These actions make it likely the FDA would also categorize cybrids as more than minimally manipulated biological products.

Cells derived from cybrids in preclinical research would also fall under the FDA's oversight for xenotransplantation. Under FDA rules biological products are the products of xenotransplantation if they are human cells "that have had ex vivo contact with live nonhuman animal cells" (Halme and Kessler 2006, 1730). In general, biological products combining human and nonhuman cells could be risky if, among other things, infectious agents passed to humans or if nonpathogenic infectious agents in humans recombined with viruses to produce new pathogenic agents (Scott 2006, 1–2). The FDA has indicated it would subject cells derived from human ES-cell lines that were cultured on animal feeder cells to testing as "stem-cell-based products." Those who produce cellular and tissue-based products must show that the products are "safe, pure, and potent" before proceeding with clinical trials (Halme and Kessler 2006, 1731–32). For ES cells the products could be stem cells that will differentiate after transfer, cells that have already differentiated, or a mixture of differentiated and undifferentiated stem cells (1730).

In the United Kingdom policy adjustments have been made for cybrids. Although the HFE Act 1990 did not mention the transfer of human nuclei to animal eggs, the question was subsequently raised. In 2000 a report from the Chief Medical Officer's Expert Group on stem cell research recommended allowing SCNT research but not the "mixing of human adult (somatic) cells with the live eggs of any animal species" (U.K. Department of Health 2000a; U.K. House of Commons 2007, 17). When Parliament revised the HFE Act in 2001 to allow therapeutic SCNT research (in response to the Expert Group's recommendation that licenses for embryo research should be extended to include research on disease and treatment), it left the question of iSCNT unaddressed (U.K. House of Commons 2007, 9). In 2004 the government announced it would review the HFE Act, and it launched a public consultation in late 2005. One matter for deliberation was whether to permit creating "human-animal hybrid or chimera embryos for research" (U.K. House of Commons 2007, 12).

In 2006 two research teams applied for licenses to use animal eggs in SCNT research (Human Fertilisation and Embryology Authority 2007a). One would use rabbit eggs and human nuclei to get ES-like cells from the SCNT process, and the other would use nuclei from somatic cells of persons with a mutation for a heart condition and pig eggs (Centre for Stem Cell Biology n.d.; Clinical Sciences Research Institute n.d.). The

SCNT process would be used to retrieve ES cells with the eventual goal of producing an ES-cell line that models a human disease (Clinical Sciences Research Institute n.d.). On December 14, 2006, the government issued its proposed revisions to the HFE Act in a White Paper. It recommended that the "creation of hybrid and chimera embryos in vitro should not be allowed." It also recommended that the revised law contain a provision to enable regulations in the future for the creation of such embryos "under licence, for research purposes only" (quoted in United Kingdom. House of Commons 2007, 13).

The HFEA, with its status as "independent regulator," conducted its own consultation (U.K. House of Commons 2007, 38). Interpreting the government's two-part recommendation (forbid but leave the door open) as restrictive, the Science and Technology Committee of the House of Commons in January 2007 started its own inquiry and advised in a March 2007 report that Parliament revise the HFE Act to provide permissive regulatory coverage of the creation of human-animal hybrid and chimera embryos (44). Another step toward this goal came in May 2008, when the House of Commons defeated by a 336–176 vote an amendment to the pro-posed revisions that would have prohibited the creation of all "admixed embryos," including cybrids (Henderson and Elliott 2008). The HFEA subsequently funded the two (and eventually additional) research proto-cols. The revised HFE Act 2008 allows the creation of admixed embryos but prohibits their transfer to a woman for procreation.

Policy advisory groups in other nations have also engaged in reviews of research using cybrids. In Australia the Lockhart Legislation Review Committee in 2005 supported the use of animal eggs for "research, train-ing and clinical application, including the production of human embry-onic stem cells" and recommended that it be allowable under license if criteria were followed, no embryos were transferred, and the entity was not allowed to develop beyond fourteen days (Legislation Review Committee 2005, 172). In late 2006 the government acted on most of the committee's recommendations but did not allow the creation of hybrid or chimera embryos. In the same legislation the government al-lowed research, under license, of therapeutic cloning (Parliament of the Commonwealth 2006a, 2006b). The vote on the bill was divided, and the restriction on creating cybrids was added to the House version following a close Senate vote the month before (Australia Approves 2006). The law had the effect of repealing a 2002 law that had forbidden the creation of cloned embryos for research purposes.

Both Canada and France bar cybrid research. Germany and Italy bar it by way of forbidding the creation of embryos for research. Austria, Norway, and Tunisia bar embryo research even on spare donated embryos (BBC News 2007). Canada's Assisted Human Reproduction Act of 2004 defines a hybrid as, in part, "an ovum of a non-human life form into which the nucleus of a human cell has been introduced" (Canada/ Government 2004). The law forbids "creat[ing] a hybrid for the purpose of reproduction" or transferring it to a human or nonhuman uterus. The law also denies a license to "create an in vitro embryo for any purpose other than creating a human being" or aiding assisted reproductive technologies (Canada/Government 2004, 5.1.a).

CROSS-SPECIES EMBRYO TRANSFER

Cross-species embryo transfer involving human and nonhuman species is exceedingly remote. The idea of transferring a nonhuman embryo to a human uterus for research or procreation is, as far as this author knows, not supported by scientific justification, and proposals are not extant about transferring a human embryo to a nonhuman uterus for research or procreation. Nevertheless cross-species embryo transfers reappear in policy deliberations. The Warnock Commission concluded years ago that placing a human embryo into an animal uterus would be "cause for concern," but it did not give reasons for recommending it be a criminal offense (U.K. House of Commons 2005, 34). In the United States the President's Council on Bioethics (PCB) in 2004 recommended that Congress pass a law to "prohibit the transfer, for any purpose, of any human embryo into the body of any member of a nonhuman species" (President's Council on Bioethics 2004, 221). It also recommended that a "bright line" be drawn at the insertion of ex vivo human embryos into the bodies of animals: "an ex vivo human embryo entering a uterus belongs *only* in a *human* uterus. If these lines should be crossed, it should only be after clear public deliberation and assent, not by the private decision of some adventurous or renegade researchers" (220).

Among countries with related laws, China stipulates that no human embryo used for research is to be transferred to "human or other animal's reproductive system" (Asia n.d.), and Japan disallows placement of human-animal interspecies embryos into a human or animal uterus (Hinxton Group 2008). Australia, Korea, and Singapore explicitly bar transferring a human embryo to an animal body and/or transferring an animal embryo to a human body (Hinxton Group 2008). Australia also forbids placing a human cloned embryo into an animal body. Some national laws also forbid placing human gametes in nonhumans or nonhuman gametes in a woman's uterus. The United Kingdom's HFE Act 2008 provides that "No person shall place in a woman a live embryo other than a human embryo" (U.K. HFE Act 2008, 3[2][a]), and "a licence cannot authorize . . . placing an embryo in any animal" (U.K. HFE Act 2008, [3][3][c]). Some regulations exist at the nongovernmental level in the United States. For example, Washington University's ESCRO stipulates that it is "not permissible" to transfer human embryos or embryos with ES cells added to a nonhuman uterus (Washington University 2005).

At present, no scientifically tenable proposals are on the table for cross-species embryo transfer involving humans. As stated in the United Kingdom "No one involved in this type of research [chimeric or cybrid embryos] is suggesting that such early stage embryos be implanted into any type of uterus, be it animal or human. . . . This procedure is viewed by the scientific community purely as a tool for the derivation of stem cells for research" (United Kingdom. Parliament 2007e). The Science and Technology Committee of the U.K. House of Commons addressed placing a human embryo in an animal uterus, and it advised not to avoid "difficult subjects which may widely be considered 'taboo'" such as this. It saw no scientific justification at present but considered a situation in which such a process might be beneficial: It is "conceivable that such research could yield valuable insights into the causes of infertility and miscarriage" (U.K. House of Commons 2007, 34). The norms of embryo research direct that human embryos "should never be used frivolously for research purposes," but incubating a human embryo in an animal's uterus might be appropriate, according to the committee, if it yielded valuable information about infertility. The committee saw no scientific justification for this at present, but if the situation arose, Parliament would be the body to consider whether to lift the current prohibitions (U.K. House of Commons 2007, 35). The committee did not recommend lifting the prohibition on the reverse transfer—placing an animal embryo in a human uterus (U.K. House of Commons 2007, 35).

Thinking about Dignity

Would transferring a human embryo to an animal uterus for research contravene human dignity? The U.K. Science and Technology Committee said it was not clear what issues this would raise for the status of the human embryo (U.K. House of Commons 2007, 34). Even the PCB recommendation seemed to leave some latitude when it stated that if lines were crossed it should be "only after public deliberation and assent."

Consider one hypothetical study in which a spare embryo is donated by a couple for research and would be examined for four days in vitro to learn more about a particular aspect of development. In a second study a spare embryo is donated, but it would be examined for four days in vivo in a mouse uterus. Each couple knows the general type of research for which the embryo will be used, including, for the second couple, the interspecies element. If the first study is ethically acceptable, provided the norms of embryo research are respected, is the second study also acceptable? In other words, does the presence of an animal component in itself make the study qualitatively different (more ethically problematic) than a study not involving an animal component? Turning to the matter of dignity, would the second study be more of an affront to human dignity than the first if the conditions and outcome are the same except for the transfer of the embryo to be examined to a mouse uterus rather than to a glass dish? In both, the embryo will be destroyed, and in both an important research question is presumed.

Leon Kass provides one perspective: Of key importance is the embryo itself and what it is—the start of a new life—not where it is placed (President's Council on Bioethics 2003b, 2). The embryo is to be protected regardless of location. A second perspective is typified by the SCHB's concern about "demean[ing] what is fully human by degrading the life in question with animal content" (United Kingdom. Parliament 2007h). Presumably, this includes the mouse uterus as animal content. It suggests that any interspecies contact between a human embryo and an animal uterus is immoral. A third perspective is taken by the Science and Technology Committee, wherein the potential benefits of the research are of primary concern. Undeniably the idea of using an animal's uterus introduces a disconcerting element, but in the absence of much discussion about this, it is not automatically apparent that the animal uterus violates human dignity, especially if using a living system yields more valid results than using in vitro methods.

In a third hypothetical study a chimeric or cybrid embryo is transferred to a mouse uterus. From one perspective this is doubly problematic (creating a chimeric or cybrid embryo and using an animal uterus). From another perspective it is less problematic because the entity is twice removed from being a viable embryo (cybrid or chimera and inhospitable uterus). At issue is how close the embryo is to being viable. Again dignity does not appear to be a more effective objection than reference to norms of embryo research. These norms place on researchers the burden to demonstrate the need for the studies and the careful articulation of harms and benefits in order to justify the study.

A fourth hypothetical scenario is to transfer a viable human embryo to a primate uterus. The rationale for this hypothetical scenario would presumably be to create conditions more compatible with a human system. The ISSCR advised against studies in which "human totipotent or pluripotent cells are implanted into a human or non-human primate uterus...at this time because of an absent international consensus about a compelling scientific rationale to do so and because of the 'strong ethical concerns' it raises" (ISSCR 2006, 7). For this research an array of objections, including a repugnance objection, would surely be raised. These objections (e.g., no justifiable reason, the need to protect two high species, less onerous alternatives, no consensus) arguably have a more persuasive empirically based weight than challenges based on human dignity objections.

A fifth hypothetical scenario has received policy attention. Here human ES cells are transferred to a mouse embryo to yield a chimeric mouse with human cells alongside mouse cells. Some of the ES cells differentiate to gametes, however, and the mouse ends up with human gametes side by side its own gametes. If a female mouse with haploid human eggs and a male mouse with haploid human sperm mated, theoretically the mating could produce a human zygote in a mouse uterus, which would be an unintentional form of human-nonhuman cross-species transfer (Board on Life Sciences and Board on Health Sciences Policy 2004, 12–13). Lee Silver turns this into a "thought experiment." Theoretically, he writes, "natural mating between such hybrid male and female mice would produce fully human embryos along with fully mouse embryos," although the mouse and human gametes could not fertilize because, among other things, humans have twenty-three pairs of chromosomes and mice have only twenty (Silver 2006, 185).

All of this is extraordinarily unlikely—not merely the inadvertent creation of human gametes from ES cells but also the capacity of the gametes to fertilize within a mouse body. Even if an embryo resulted, it would be incapable of sustained growth because of immunological barriers and because a human embryo implanted in a mouse uterus would not portend well for the mother mouse. What is at issue here is not the creation of a human-mouse hybrid but the possibility of inadvertent fertilization of a human egg by a human sperm. That possibility, however remote, was enough for the ISSCR, NAS, and NIH in its draft guidelines to recommend that "animal chimeras incorporating human cells with the potential to form gametes" should not be allowed to produce offspring, either naturally or in vitro (ISSCR 2006, 7). According to the ISSCR, "interbreeding of such chimeras should not be allowed, to preclude the possibility of inadvertent human-human fertilization events" (7).

The reverse move—transferring animal embryos to a human uterus—lacks justification and would pose risks of viral contamination, immunological rejection, and inadvertent implantation. If the plan were to remove the uterus in any event (e.g., a scheduled hysterectomy), it would still not be acceptable because of the absence of a compelling reason and the presence of exploitative elements. Risky research violates the respect due to participants.

Thinking about Procreation

Would cross-species embryo transfer lead to procreation? The HERP over a decade expressed overwhelming sentiment against transferring a human embryo to an animal uterus for procreation (National Institutes of Health 1994, 96). The members cited the great risk of rejection or changes

to maternal-fetal placental interactions, risks to children, "scientific inva-
lidity," and moral opposition. According to the HERP, the maternal-fetal
interaction is physiological and psychological, and it would be "repugnant" to experiment with a relationship between a human fetus and a
nonhuman gestational mother. This would be extremely risky (if not impossible) for the developing fetus and animal surrogate, most likely a nonhuman primate. Among other things the placental tissue of the mother
and fetus would not match, and the size of the uterine space would be at
odds with fetal size. It would raise "clear issues of animal welfare" (U.K.
House of Commons 2007, 34).

The reverse move—transferring an animal embryo to a woman's uterus
for the purpose of procreation—would be incredibly risky to the woman
and have no justification. No conceivable reason exists to put a woman
into the position of being a surrogate mother to a nonhuman animal even
if this were physiologically possible. Moreover, public sentiment against
either type of surrogacy would be distinctly hostile. Even E. B. White, the
author of *Stuart Little*, had to appease his editor by revising his opening
page to clarify that Stuart the mouse had been adopted by the Littles and
not born to Mrs. Little (Sagoff 2007, 51).

Policy Directions

In the HFE Act of 1990 the United Kingdom forbade placing a "live
embryo other than a human embryo" or any "live gametes other than
human gametes" in a woman even though policy makers acknowledge
there is no reason for conducting such tests (U.K. Department of Health
2006, 22; U.K. House of Commons 2007, 50). The Act also stated that
research licenses would not be granted to place a human embryo into an
animal (Human Genetics Advisory Committee 1998, 34). The Science
and Technology Committee recommended that "legislation prohibit the
implantation of human-animal chimera or hybrid embryos in a woman"
(U.K. House of Commons 2007, 34). The HFE Act 2008 bars transfer
of any nonpermitted gametes or embryos (including nonhuman) to a
woman's uterus. It also bars transfer of human admixed embryos to an
animal.

In Australia the Prohibition of Human Cloning for Reproduction and
the Regulation of Human Embryo Research Amendment Act of 2006 pro-

hibited placing a human embryo clone into a human or an animal body, placing a human embryo in an animal body, or placing an animal embryo into a human body "for any period of gestation" (U.K. Department of Health 2007a, Appendix C). In Canada the Assisted Human Reproduction Act of 2004 barred a variety of cross-species transfers, including placing a human embryo clone into a human or any "non-human life form," transferring a nonhuman life form (sperm, egg, embryo, or fetus) to a human being, or transferring a chimera or hybrid into a human or "non-human life form" (U.K. Department of Health 2007a, Appendix C). Singapore's Human Cloning and Other Prohibited Practices Act 2004 forbids placing a cloned human embryo into a human or animal body (Hinxton Group 2008). Japanese law states that "No person shall transfer a human somatic clone embryo, a human-animal amphimictic embryo, a human-hybrid embryo or a human-animal chimeric embryo into the uterus of a human or an animal" (Law Concerning Regulation Relating to Human Cloning Techniques and Other Similar Techniques [Law No. 146 2000]; Hinxton Group 2008).

One justification for using a legal ban to prevent interspecies embryo transfer rather than voluntary restrictions is to create a clean line between research and procreation. If procreation is of concern, then forbidding the transfer of an embryo from one species to another addresses that concern and enables other forms of ISR to proceed. Barring the transfer is simpler than trying to guess motive, as one is left to do with a law that bans the creation of a cybrid or chimera for the "purpose of procreation."

The underlying tone of such restrictions also is informative. The "egregious research" approach that targets human-animal hybrids and embryo transfer conveys skepticism about the trustworthiness of scientists. The United Kingdom follows a crisper approach that includes embryo transfer in a broader regulatory framework as it tries to anticipate a variety of research endeavors that may require regulation. As one British scientist observed "It is far better to control such research activities under a good regulatory system through careful consideration of proposed experiments by scientific and ethical review panels, than it is by prohibitive laws that are likely to be both too restrictive and leave dangerous loopholes, especially in this rapidly advancing field of science" (United Kingdom.

Parliament 2007f). On the other hand, restrictions on speculative techniques are necessarily based on a sketchy understanding of what may be done, when, and why.

TRANSGENICS

The artist Eduardo Kac famously arranged for the conception and birth of Alba, an albino rabbit born in France in 2000 after having been injected as a single-cell fertilized egg with the green fluorescent gene from the jellyfish *Aequorea victoria* (Kac [2000]). As a result of the genetic alteration, Alba glowed green when viewed under a special blue light. She lived with Kac and his family and was a regular rabbit except for the jellyfish gene in all her body cells. Kac actively promoted Alba as a form of living art and wrote a book in homage: *It's Not Easy Being Green!* Kac used transgenic art to illustrate the "fluidity of the concept of species" in a culture that he regarded as increasingly transgenic.

A transgenic animal such as Alba is one in which sequences of foreign DNA have been added to the genome. These sequences are introduced into the organism's germ line by, for example, injecting DNA from another organism into a single-cell embryo (Witherly, Perry, and Leja 2001, 121). A transgene (cross gene) may be a complete gene sequence from another organism, a sequence synthesized in vitro, or a combination. In brief: "A transgenic animal is an animal which has been genetically modified by the stable incorporation, by using artificial gene transfer, of exogenous DNA into its genome, in order to introduce or delete specific characteristics of the phenotype" (ECVAM Workshop 28 n.d., 2). If DNA is "stably incorporated" into the animal's genotype, then the animal and its offspring "will possess an altered phenotype" (Singleton 2000, 1090). The animals will have a "desired genetic property" that expresses "novel phenotypes" (1090). Because the DNA was recombined at the germ line, the modification will be inherited. Genetically altered animals have many uses, including the development of animal models for human diseases and the production of pharmaceuticals.

Investigators first successfully created genetically altered mice in 1980 by splicing DNA fragments from one organism into fragments from another organism to create a recombinant DNA molecule that could be inserted into the germ line. Transgenic research allows the spread of a gene within a species at a faster rate than would have occurred naturally, and it can be intra- or interspecific. If the latter, it is, loosely speaking, a form of ISR, and the recipient will express genetic information not usually found in its own species (Singleton 2000, 1090).

Transgenic animals with one or more human-like genes are commonly used in research to study gene activity and to make animal models of human diseases (United Kingdom. Parliament 2007f). Transgenics enables researchers to study gene expression in the whole animal, which is a more realistic setting because diseases generally involve interactions among different types of cells (Witherly, Perry, and Leja 2001, 121).

An organism's genome can also be altered by a knockout method, which is distinct from the knock-in method described above. Here, part of the organism's genome is disabled at the gametic or embryonic stage so the animal will lack the capability related to that gene or genes (Nuffield Council on Bioethics 2005, 5.18). This furthers knowledge about the function of that gene or genes, and it is a method for creating animal models of human disease. Interspecies splicing can be animal-animal, human-animal, or, theoretically, animal-human. An example of animal-animal transgenics is to splice spider genes to goat embryos so the spider genes will express a protein for silk in the goats' mammary glands, which then appears in the goats' milk. This silk is stronger than silk from worms, and using the milk is an easier way to secure the silk protein than to harvest silk from spiders naturally.

Human-nonhuman transgenics creates animals that express human proteins in milk, muscles, and other places. For example, transgenic chickens express human proteins in their egg whites for pharmaceutical use, and goats have been altered to express a human protein in their milk to induce thickening of blood (Alper 2003; Transgenic Drug 2006). Researchers have been creating mouse transgenic models for human disease for over twenty years (U.K. Department of Health 2007a, Appendix H. 3.8). Human data are used to refine mouse models and develop therapies. Mouse cells and tissues are likely increasingly to resemble human cells and tissues as research proceeds (Dennis 2006, 741).

Transgenics studies do not attract the same level of wariness as other forms of early ISR reviewed in this book. The report of the U.K. Science and Technology Committee, for example, briefly included transgenics in its discussion of hybrids and chimeras, noting that "transgenic animals are not routinely referred to as 'hybrids' but do contain a mix of DNA" (U.K. House of Commons 2007, 20). Transgenic research is also apropos because knockout genetic technologies are used to create chimeras. Moreover, gene splicing between human and nonhuman is a likelier way to integrate human-nonhuman biological processes than by creation of hybrids or chimeras.

Thinking about Dignity

Does splicing human DNA sequences into the genomes of nonhuman animals for research purposes violate human dignity? Is the splicing of individual genes or gene fragments different from the more significant integration of human and nonhuman DNA that would occur with hybrids? How much genetic material does it take to make a dignity argument? Gene splicing is done, as noted above, for the study of human disease and for various commercial goals. The National Council of Churches in the United States opposes the creation of human-nonhuman chimeras, but in a document about biotechnologies it indicated it would not foreclose "minimal gene transfers between species" if these would "result in clear evidence of realizable medical benefits" and if a "thorough public debate" were carried out, including participation by religious leaders, in search of a consensus (National Council of Churches n.d., 9). In the United Kingdom, the Christian Action Research and Education Group, which is opposed to most early IRS, accepts inserting one human gene into another species. It does not accept alterations that would "cause observable changes in the resulting transgenic animal" or "produce observable human characteristics" (United Kingdom. Parliament 2007i). The group is more cautious "the more we cross the species barrier" and is concerned about what "percentage of human genes make an animal more than just an animal and what percentage of animal genes make a human less than human?" (United Kingdom. Parliament 2007i). Other observers also believe that inserting human genes into the genomes of nonhumans should "only proceed with extreme caution" and "may be undertaken for preventive, diagnostic or therapeutic purposes and only if its aim is not to introduce any modifications in the genome of descendants" (United Kingdom. Parliament 2007c).

A dignity argument is not powerful here because a limited number of genes is not equated with humanness. Introducing segments of DNA from the human genome into an animal is not consequential for humans. Gene transfers are targeted to biological functions and the expression of proteins, not to personal attributes. The Boyd Group, an interdisciplinary group reporting on genetically modified animals, has written: "Talk of 'mixing' genomes does not reflect the nature of genetic engineering as currently practiced. Although there is a random element, present practice usually involves the relatively precise transfer of only one or two genes. . . . Each gene codes for a specific protein, and it is only the combined effects of expression of a multitude of genes within the living organism that confer, say, its 'pig-ness' or its 'human-ness.' Furthermore, many genes are conserved (are similar) between different species" (Boyd Group 1999, 5).

Would the reverse transfer—splicing nonhuman genes into human embryos for research—violate human dignity? The U.K. Department of Health sees no proposals to do this at present but could envision it to study gene function in early embryos or to introduce a gene that would make it easier to derive ES cells (U.K. Department of Health 2007a, Appendix B. 1.2.1). If the resulting entity is studied and then destroyed, following the norm that human embryos subject to nontherapeutic research must not be transferred for procreation, then the same rules apply as for chimeric research. In some ways resistance to this research takes on the tone of genetic exceptionalism, in which the mere presence of genes is thought to provoke qualitatively unique issues. It is hard to see, however, how splicing "non-human animal" genes for research purposes would be more injurious to human dignity than the insertion of newly created synthetic genes or chromosomes.

Thinking about Procreation

Would the ability to manipulate the human genome in the laboratory by splicing in, say, genes associated with an animal's night vision, lead to the transfer of manipulated embryos for procreation? Lively debate accompanies questions about the ethics of modifying the human germ line, and the question of splicing "animal genes" such as those that improve visual acuity to human embryos would fall under deliberations about inheritable genetic modifications (IGMs), with enhancement alterations in particular. As some are exploring, defending, or even endorsing human IGMs (see, e.g., Walters and Palmer 1997; Buchanan et al. 2000; Frankel and Chapman 2000; Stock 2002; Chapman and Frankel 2003; Savulescu 2003; Genetics and Public Policy Center 2005; Allhoff 2005; Harris 2007), as germ line alterations with animals proceed briskly, and as the genomes of an increasing number of species are mapped and sequenced, it is not unrealistic to suppose that research about IGMs for humans is on the horizon. Again, however, this research will not likely involve literally splicing animal genes to human embryos. Instead synthetic genes and long stretches of DNA, perhaps modeled after animal genes, more likely will be used (Biologists Weigh Up 2005; Endy 2005). "Animalness" is not the issue here; at issue rather are the purpose and implications of the research (Savulescu and Skene 2008). To focus on nonhuman-human gene transfer as a technique is to miss the larger set of issues associated with enhancement technologies.

Thinking about Species

Transgenic research has spawned a particularly rich imagery in art and literature. According to Philip Reilly, "transgenics, our ability to move genes across species barriers, has held great allure for artists" (Anker and Nelkin 2004, xiv). For example, the 2002 photographic exhibit, *Genesis*, featured realistic faces of people with blended animal and human features to become Leopard Spirit, Horse Face, and other singular creations (Random Samples 2002). Similarly, Dean Koontz's novel, *Watchers*, features Einstein, a lovable transgenic golden retriever with human-like intelligence. The dog was created, says one of the book characters, by "inserting that foreign genetic material into the retriever's genetic code, simultaneously editing out the dog's own genes that limited its intelligence to that of a dog" (Koontz 1987, 223). The same scientists who produced Einstein also created his evil opposite, the murderous "Outsider," with the brute strength of an orangutan and the cunning of a human. Transgenics provokes thinking about blending between species, but because it has heretofore involved mostly animal-animal splicing, its interspecies dimensions have not attracted significant policy attention outside of protections accorded animals in research.

Transgenics does have a significant impact on animals, however. For one thing the studies use a large number of animals. Observers in the United Kingdom reported that the overall use of laboratory animals declined somewhat between 1990 and 1996, reflecting deliberate efforts to reduce the number of animals used, but the number of animals used in genetic research increased by 525 percent (ECVAM Workshop 28 n.d., 7). This growth offset reductions in the use of animals for other purposes such as toxicology testing (Abbott 1999).

A committee from the United Kingdom's House of Lords also found that the number of animals used in research remained stable except for a "dramatic" increase in genetically modified animals (United Kingdom. Parliament 2002, 1). The committee reported that in 1995, 8 percent of the total number of procedures were on genetically modified animals, but that figure had risen to 21 percent in 2000 (1).

It is reasonable to expect genome studies to lead to even greater increases in the number of animals, particularly mice. In the United States the Knockout Mouse Project aims to produce ten types of mutants for each of the ten thousand to thirty thousand genes in the mouse genome (Grimm 2006, 1862; NIH Cash 2006). The eventual goal is to develop hundreds of thousands of mouse lines corresponding to diseases in humans. The counterparts to the U.S. project include the European Conditional Knockout Mouse Mutagenesis program and the North American Conditional Knockout Mouse Mutagenesis program (Qui 2006, 814).

At least three hundred thousand new lines could be developed over the next couple of decades (Abbott 2004). It will take, by one calculation, fifty to several hundred mice to establish a line for one gene and then several hundred more for genetic and phenotypic analysis of that line (Qui 2006, 814). With at least twenty-five thousand genes in the mouse genome, this points to seven million mice for the project. Ideally, mouse embryos will be recorded in repositories and frozen and shipped as potential breeding pairs to researchers internationally. Embryo freezing and shipping prevents wear and tear on adult mice, and it lessens expenses and space requirements for storing live mice. If a line is not in a public repository, however, other researchers may unnecessarily replicate the line. A survey conducted by the U.S. National Institutes of Health revealed that only one-quarter of knockout lines created are in public repositories.

Over seven hundred lines have been created more than three times (Qui 2006, 815).

Another reason to suppose continued growth in the number of research mice is the advance of stem-cell science. As research moves closer to clinical trials, animal models will be used to evaluate safety and efficacy prior to research using human participants (BVAAWF 2003). Rodents have been a central part of ES-cell science for several decades. In the 1960s and 1970s investigators studied the properties of mouse embryonal carcinoma cells and in 1981 reported the derivation of ES cells from the inner cell mass of mouse embryos (Roussant 2004, xxi). Thus developments in stem-cell science "have made mouse ES cells an incredibly powerful tool" for altering a mouse's genome and studying the effects (xii).

Investigators create mouse chimeras to develop genetic lines, so chimeras and transgenics can be discussed in tandem. The welfare of the animals used in transgenic research is affected in several ways. For one thing it is hard to predict where the altered gene or DNA sequence will land in the embryonic genome (Boyd Group 1999, 8). Insertional mutations can result when DNA lands in or near a functioning gene, so each animal is experimental for both the expected and unexpected impacts of the intervention. Consequently, "each transgenic founder animal is unique in terms of both genetic makeup and the nature of any defects resulting from insertional mutations" (ECVAM Workshop n.d.). The use of ES cells may reduce this uncertainty if the technology enables more precise targeting of gene insertion.

The intervention also affects animal welfare when the transgene is expressed. The severity of the impact depends on a number of factors, such as the biological properties of the target protein, where in the body the transgenes are expressed, and the degree of expression of the transgene. At one end of the spectrum, the animal could have "inert proteins . . . synthesised at a low level in a limited number of specific tissues insulated from the bloodstream." At the other end the animal could have "a condition in which a biologically highly active protein is synthesised in large amounts in many tissues with abundant access to the bloodstream" (ECVAM Workshop n.d., 12).

An example of the latter is the "Beltsville pig," which was genetically modified as an embryo at the USDA research center in Beltsville, MD to produce human growth hormone (McKibben 2003, 40–41). Although the primary goal was achieved—the pig produced human growth hormone—the intervention had unanticipated impacts on the pig's metabolism. One person observed that the pig was "excessively hairy, lethargic, riddled with arthritis, apparently impotent, and slightly cross-eyed . . . [and] the pig could hardly stand up" (41). With genetic modifications, as with cloning, the impact may not be known for years. Moreover, one gets a "'sudden' introduction of a distant gene in a new organism," which contrasts to traditional methods of selective breeding that reveal problems at an earlier stage and enable corrective action (Nuffield Council on Bioethics 2005, 3.41). A report from Denmark indicated that 21 percent of strains of genetically modified animals experienced minor discomfort, 30 percent experienced increases in mortality and disease, and 15 percent experienced severe discomfort (Nuffield Council on Bioethics 2005, 4.57).

With the large range of genetic modification studies, there is no simple picture of the well-being of genetically altered animals because the impact depends on which genes are altered or knocked out. The impact could be virtually nil, or it could be severe, as in a mouse born without a growth factor receptor gene that leaves the mouse with severe skeletal defects or other major abnormalities (Nuffield Council on Bioethics 2005, 5.22). In addition not all mutations show themselves in a clear way. These uncertainties will affect the Knockout Mouse Project, where researchers will know little or nothing about the function of many of the mouse genes and will be unable to predict what will happen when the genes are inactivated (Grimm 2006, 1862). In short, mutation studies have unpredictable and variable impacts on animal welfare.

Genetic alterations can also cause premature death indirectly through microinjection or transfer of embryos destined to become larger than normal fetuses to surrogate mice of regular size (ECVAM Workshop n.d., 11). The method of creating transgenic animals can also matter, as indicated in a study comparing mice modified by injection into the pronucleus of a fertilized egg with ES-cell-mediated gene transfer (van der Meer 2002). The author found that mice born following both methods had greater mortality and body weight than control mice and that 8 percent of the ES-cell-mediated mice were hermaphrodites. She noticed no observable effects on development or behavior. She developed a scoring system to measure intended and unintended effects of transgenics. A report from the United Kingdom's House of Lords on the Animals in Scientific Procedures of 2002 likewise recommended that all new strains of transgenic animals receive a welfare assessment "as a matter of course" (United Kingdom. Parliament 2002, 2).

Inefficiencies contribute to the large number of animals used for breeding to produce each strain (Nuffield Council on Bioethics 2005, 5.22). Most embryos do not survive the intervention, and only a few (1–30 percent) of those that survive to birth actually have the intended modification—an average success rate of 15 percent (ECVAM Workshop n.d., S1–S3). It has been estimated that to produce two to eight transgenic mice, 300–350 eggs are injected with the gene in question. From these, twenty to fifty live mice will be born, and only two to eight will have the transgene (Animal Testing n.d., 4). Creating chimeric mice also involves wastage. If ES cells are injected into 150–175 mouse blastocysts, thirty to fifty live mice will be born, and two to six of them will have sufficient fur color mottling to indicate "a good chance for embryonic stem cell contribution to the germline" (Animal Testing n.d., 4).

Policy Directions
The "three R policy," first articulated in the United Kingdom in 1959 and recognized in the United States and other countries, aims to reduce the number of animals used in research, refine experimental procedures so they are less onerous for the animals, and replace animals wherever possible through computer simulations or the use of human cells and tissues (Russell and Burch 1992). The United Kingdom has a relatively thorough policy regarding animals in research, as illustrated by the establishment in 2004 of the National Centre for the Replacement, Refinement and Reduction of Animals, an independent center funded by the government, Wellcome Trust, and research corporations. The three R policy is now "widely accepted internationally as criteria for humane animal use in research and testing" (National Centre n.d.).

The first R, replacement, means pursuing scientific goals through methods that do not use living animals (Nuffield Council on Bioethics

2005, 190). Replacement is complete if it relies on "physical and chemical properties of molecules, mathematical and computer studies of biological processes" or human cells and tissues solely. It is incomplete if it uses some biological material from animals for cell culture and where the animals are kept alive or killed humanely (191). The second R, refinement, aims for less severe procedures and improved animal welfare. It includes minimizing pain, using smaller needles, refining endpoints, and killing animals as early and humanely as possible (212). Animal welfare can be improved by studying the behavior of animals to determine what helps them flourish (211–12).

The third R, reduction, limits the number of animals in research without subjecting the remaining animals to more experiments (Nuffield Council on Bioethics 2005, 206). Reduction can be achieved by using appropriate statistical designs, sharing negative research findings to avoid duplication of studies, and coordinating international regulations so studies need not be repeated in different countries (205, 207). Most important, however, is to question the need for conducting the study at all and to ask whether the experiment is worth pain and suffering for the animal (194). As reiterated by the Boyd Group, "whenever animals are genetically modified and used in science, there should be careful, detailed and critical scrutiny of the consequences of that use, and serious, honest reflection on the need to use animals at all" (Boyd Group 1999, 13).

A workshop to study the use of transgenic animals in the European Union recommended that transgenic animals be monitored on a case-by-case basis because each founder animal is unique (ECVAM Workshop n.d.). The group endorsed previous recommendations that a "genuine social need" must exist before new transgenic strains are created and that "technological opportunity" is not enough to justify creating these lines. The group held the use of primates in transgenic work to be unacceptable in principle (19).

Policy related to inheritable genetic modifications in humans is nearly nonexistent in the United States, where the National Institutes of Health "Points to Consider" document states that the Recombinant DNA Advisory Committee (RAC) and its Working Group on Human Gene Therapy "will not at present entertain proposals for germ line alterations"

(National Institutes of Health 1985). This does not forbid research into human IGMs in privately financed work, but it forecloses federal funding of such studies and reduces the opportunity for the RAC to deliberate about inheritable modifications.

Other countries have a variety of limitations on germ line altera- tions. In Canada the Assisted Human Reproduction Act of 2004 pro- hibits "altering the genome of a cell of a human being or in vitro embryo such that the alteration is capable of being transmitted to descendants." Australia, Germany, the United Kingdom, Israel, and South Africa are among at least ten countries that also prohibit germ line gene therapy (U.K. Department of Health 2007a, Appendix C; Fukuyama and Furger 2006, 403–5). The United Kingdom forbids transferring a "human em- bryo that has been altered by the introduction of any sequence of nuclear or mitochondrial DNA of an animal into one or more cells of the embryo" (U.K. HFE Act 2008, Part 1.3(2)(6)(c)).

SUMMARY

This chapter deals with three types of early ISR. The first, the creation of cybrids through iSCNT, would in its present iteration be used pri- marily to extract human ES cells. In 1998 researchers at Advanced Cell Therapeutics announced that they had combined human somatic cell nuclei with cow eggs and that the entities had cleaved before the researchers destroyed them. This, along with the announcement by Chinese researchers in 2003 that they had fused human nuclei with rabbit eggs, amounted to focusing events that drew attention to the ethics of iSCNT. The benefits of such research would be significant in light of a shortage of human eggs. President Clinton's request to the NBAC in 1998 to consider the ethical implications of using animal eggs in SCNT research briefly made cybrids a policy matter, but the issue faded from public view in the United States after the NBAC issued a short report saying that not enough information existed to draw conclusions about the ethics of using animal eggs.

Later, when two research teams in the United Kingdom submitted protocols involving cybrids to the HFE Act, they set the stage for a particular policy question, namely, whether cybrids were embryos under the auspices of the HFE Act. The determination that they did fall under the regulatory framework of the HFE Act allowed research to proceed with careful scrutiny. In the United Kingdom experience, cybrids were a live policy matter with deliberations grounded by reasonably imminent science and realistic rationales. A claim that the creation of cybrids for research violates human dignity is not backed by persuasive arguments that the cybrid technique is fundamentally different from other forms of research using embryos. In fact the impact on dignity may be less if the cybrid cannot be viable.

Nor are procreation arguments persuasive; no rationale exists for using animal eggs for human procreation when human eggs are available. Reputable researchers are not interested in pursuing reproductive SCNT, much less iSCNT. Species-confusion arguments are unpersuasive because the cybrid genome would be distinctly human; the nonhuman animal would contribute cytoplasm only. Although cytoplasm is essential for cell function, substituting animal for human cytoplasm would not directly affect the nuclear genes linked to social and intellectual capabilities attributed to humans.

Human-nonhuman and nonhuman-human embryo transfers are also remote. They do not amount to live ethical or policy problems inasmuch as they lack focusing events, research protocols, advocates, and rationales. The idea of cross-species embryo transfer is odd in light of the alternative of in vitro environments. The impact of cross-species embryo transfer as a metaphor for unbridled technology is evident in proposals to ban animal-human and human-animal embryo transfers. A disjuncture exists, however, between the severe restrictions (banning) and the remoteness of the threat. An animal embryo is not likely to be transferred to a woman's uterus in the foreseeable future, if ever, which renders the rationale behind preemptive bans curious.

Transgenics is already widely practiced with animals carrying human genes in research and development. Splicing human DNA and inserting it into the germ line of the animal allows researchers to study how genes express in a living system. Although nonhuman-human transgenics is not a live issue, the prospect of genetic modifications for humans is. The issues raised by inheritable genetic modifications relate to the outcome, however, not to the source of the genes. Using nonhuman animal genes is not significantly different from using synthetic genes or chromosomes if the prospect of genetic alteration is the overall concern.

Chapter 4

Beliefs about Interspecies Interventions

WHY DOES EARLY INTERSPECIES RESEARCH (ISR) matter? What accounts for the animus by some and largely silent acceptance by others? Understanding some of the bases for conflicting views helps indicate how early ISR is political in the way it attracts attention, elicits emotion, and prompts action to protect values thought to be threatened. Of the many beliefs that animate the matter of early ISR, four are considered in this chapter: (1) orientation toward biotechnology, (2) acceptance of intuitive reactions, (3) trust in ability to draw lines, and (4) belief in firmness of the line between human and nonhuman animals.

ORIENTATION TO BIOTECHNOLOGY

Biotechnology refers to the use of "biological systems, living organisms, or derivatives thereof, to make or modify products or processes for specific use" (Rifkin 1998, 1). It is a subset of technology, which is the applied use of scientific principles and findings for human practical use (Singleton 2000, 1088). Biotechnology dates at least from times when humans began planting crops and noticed that some seeds produced better crops than others (Silver 2006, 259). By selectively using seeds from crops that were superior in some ways, humans manipulated biological processes for their own benefit. They also did so by combining grains and yeasts to produce alcohol, cross-breeding dogs to produce animals for specific uses, and catapulting bodies with bubonic plague over the walls of fortified medieval towns to spread toxins that would cause the deaths of people in the enemy community (Derbes 1966).

Biotechnology includes a range of activities such as creating vaccines, altering corn genetically to resist insects, creating mouse models of human disease, and manufacturing artificial blood. Its use accelerated in the twentieth century, particularly after the first published instance of recombinant DNA (r-DNA) research in 1973 and the subsequent application of this technique for microorganisms, plants, animals, and humans. An early example of r-DNA work in plants occurred in the 1980s with the planned introduction of a bacterium, known as ice minus, into strawberry plants to increase their resistance to frost. The first recombinant mouse was created in 1974, and this was followed in 1980 by the first patented mammal, Oncomouse, which was genetically altered to grow tumors more quickly than ordinary mice in order to aid the study of cancer-causing agents. The first experimental use for humans of genetically modified cells was approved in 1990, when somatic cells were removed, altered, and transferred back to a young girl who had ADA deficiency. Recombinant work has come to be equated with "modern" biotechnology, which produces novel biological outcomes that could not happen with traditional selective breeding.

Biotechnology has both alluring and disconcerting dimensions. According to one observer, to be modern is "to find ourselves in an environment that promises us adventure, power, joy, growth, transformation of ourselves and the world—and, at the same time, that threatens to destroy everything we have, everything we know" (Marshall Berman, quoted in Turney 1998, 6). Some groups express skepticism about the goodness of at least some uses of biotechnology. They urge caution about releasing genetically modified organisms to the environment, where these organisms can proliferate without natural controls. Others warn of the economic impulse behind biotechnology. As one author put it, "genetic engineering biotechnology is bad science working together with big business for quick profit, against the public good, against public will and aspirations, against the moral values of society and the world community" (Ho 2000, vi). From this perspective biotechnology is dangerous because it is an "unprecedented alliance between two great powers that can make or break the world: science and commerce" (Ho 2000, 13).

Jeremy Rifkin, a vocal critic of biotechnology, sees animal-human interchanges as a particularly onerous prospect for the future: "We could also see the creation of a range of new chimeric animals on Earth, including human/animal hybrids. A chimp/hume, half chimpanzee and half human, for example, could become a reality. The human-animal hybrids could be widely used as experimental subjects in medical research and as organ 'donors' for xenotransplantation. The artificial creation and propagation of cloned, chimeric, and transgenic animals could mean the end of the wild and the substitution of a bioindustrial world" (Rifkin 1998, 2).

Some embrace the economic and public health potential of biotechnologies in general but are wary of technologies they feel will make human reproduction a commodity. In general skeptics view biotechnology as a misguided attempt to master nature, and they see the future as a slippery slope that is hard for humans to control. They also express concern about losing respect for the mysteries of nature.

For others, biotechnology promises a positive future. It beckons with prospects of drugs tailored for individual patients, crops that will thrive in deserts, vaccine-laced bananas for easy inoculation, and other benefits for human health. From this perspective biotechnology has a positive impact on public health and economic development, and it is a logical use of human tools and capacities, provoking enthusiasm about the impact of innovative biotechnology on the well-being of humans and their environment (Manning 2000). Lee Silver regards finding answers as a prized goal: "To a molecular biologist, a living organism is not the 'mystery' most theologians claim. It is simply a puzzle in which many pieces have already been fitted together" (Silver 2006, 17).

Optimists see virtues of biotechnology as including scientific discovery (and its serendipitous offshoots), international standing in science, medical therapies, and the yen to advance a modern society. Using the life sciences to promote the human condition is a celebration of human ingenuity and enterprise, and it flourishes under minimal regulatory systems. Biotechnology is associated with ambitious projects such as the Human Genome Project, the Proteome Project, the Knockout Mouse Project, and the sequencing of genomes of multiple species. From this point of view biotechnology has a positive impact on human health and prosperity. For the most part, risks are within human power to anticipate and control.

WISDOM ABOUT INTUITIVE REACTIONS

One dimension that contributes to perspectives of biotechnology is the inclination to listen to intuitive reactions. Leon Kass, for example, believes that repugnance is the "emotional expression of deep wisdom" (Kass 1997). In an oft-cited article on cloning, he wrote that "Shallow are the souls that have forgotten how to shudder." Repugnance itself is not enough to call something immoral, but it is instead "at most a pointer" (Jones 2007, 768, 771). Mary Midgley also wrote of the wisdom of emotions: "We must spell out the message of our emotions and see what they are trying to tell us" (quoted in Macklin 2006, 39). Part of listening to repugnance is to "[lift] the veil from society's most delicate implicit moral sentiments" and explore taboos (Levin 2003, 54). A taboo, writes Yuval Levin, "marks a barrier whose violation would strike so deep that we would not have the words to describe it, but we would understand such a violation fully and at once" (Levin 2003, 54). Referring to interspecies beings, he writes that "taboos stand guard at the border crossings between the realm of the properly human and those of the beasts and the gods" (Levin 2003, 55). The chimera of Greek mythology was seen as a "monstrous unnatural body [signifying] a monstrous unnatural disposition" (Karpowicz, Cohen, and van der Kooy 2005, 108). The Minotaur, a man with the head of a bull who was the result of a sexual union between the Queen of Crete, Pasiphae, and a bull, was described as a "peculiarly unfortunate creature, combining the weakness of a man with the limited intelligence and inarticulateness of a bull" (President's Council on Bioethics 2005c, 3; Bazoupoulou-Kyrkanidou 2001, 77).

Repugnance may be a reaction to something that could not happen in nature. As described by Karpowicz et al. "It is a moral good for each kind of being to be aligned with its appropriate end and a moral wrong to alter its natural functioning in ways that distort or violate this end" (Karpowicz, Cohen, and van der Kooy 2005, 113). In this view "to transfer human cells, tissues, and organs into nonhumans in ways that change their function, their progression toward their end or goal, would violate the natural teleology of these beings and therefore would be unnatural and wrong." Karpowicz et al. point out that intuitions are different from emotions. Intuitions are thought to reflect an "authoritarian inner voice" (111).

It is one thing to recognize repugnance and another to ask whether there is wisdom in that repugnance (Jones 2007, 768). Tenets of evolutionary psychology suggest that repugnance has (or had) utility. According to Leda Cosmides and John Tooby, as humans evolved they developed "neural universal reasoning circuits" that helped human ancestors resolve problems facing them (Cosmides and Tooby n.d., 3). Among these reasoning circuits were those that caused humans to react with repulsion to situations that posed dangers in the past. This reaction could surface in contemporary times as a negative reaction to something that was once wisely a taboo but that might not be relevant today. Pathways developed during evolution relied on speed to ensure quick responses to threats: "Emotionally triggered pathways thus present a real evolutionary advantage" (McDermott 2004, 698).

Rose McDermott posits that rational decision making depends on "prior emotional processing" and that emotions with an evolutionary basis (e.g., fear response for survival) can surface quickly and without prior thought (McDermott 2004, 691). According to McDermott, emotional rationality includes the supposition that "emotions can provide the basis of hunches" (700). The implication is that intuitive reactions to such things as ISR may be recognized along with rational thinking (e.g., cost/benefit calculations) for a combined intuitive-rational response. Repugnance can draw attention, but it will not necessarily prevail once cognitive processing starts. For example, in a survey conducted in the United Kingdom, respondents were asked a general question about cybrids: "To what extent do you agree or disagree with scientists creating an embryo which contains mostly human with a small amount of animal genetic material purely for research?" Nearly half of the respondents (48 percent) either strongly disagreed (27 percent) or disagreed (21 percent) with the statement. The percentage disagreeing or strongly disagreeing dropped markedly when a rationale for the research was added. Responses to the question, "to what extent do you agree or disagree with creating embryos which contain mostly human and a small amount of animal genetic material in research if it may help to understand some diseases, for example Parkinson's and motor neuron disease?" showed that only 25 percent strongly disagreed (12 percent) or disagreed (13 percent) (Human Fertilisation and Embryology Authority 2007a, Appendix F).

Although repugnance may play a role in the formation of attitudes, it is not necessarily an effective policy guide. Kass thinks one does not need a "full rational justification" for things that elicit repugnance (quoted in Cohen 2007b, 121). But Rollin asserts that it is not enough to assume that something is morally wrong: It is also essential to know why it is wrong and why it is a "legitimate moral-based response" (Rollin 2007, 645). Cohen, too, says the reasons for repugnance are what matter. Relying on emotions, of which repugnance is one, can "obscure, rather than clarify, our ethical reflections" (Cohen 2007b, 121). Reasons are needed for one's moral judgments; it is not enough simply to assert them. Moreover, what is a repulsive practice in one historical era can be legitimate in another. Some taboos fade away; they also vary from one culture to the next and "can be mistaken" (Karpowicz, Cohen, and van der Kooy 2005, 111).

If no cognitive element combines with intuition to evaluate the acceptability of a technology, writes Ruth Macklin, one is left in a "fog of feeling" (Macklin 2006, 39). Appeals to "emotion, sentiment, and intuition" are directed to morality, human dignity, and concepts that are hard to measure. If the awe humans are supposed to feel is "inarticulable," this makes it a difficult argument to refute (Macklin 2006, 37). Hans Jonas's legacy lives here, R. Alta Charo asserts, as he endorsed a "heuristics of fear" using science fiction stories in bioethics in order to present "a threat to the image of man to assure ourselves of his true image by the very recoil from these threats" (Charo 2004, 308). Using repulsion to stop developments in biotechnology does not encourage reasoned discourse about what is worrisome and what can be done to address concerns. Avoiding the use of repulsion as the basis of decision making includes avoiding "outrageous scenarios that elicit emotion even while straining credulity" (Jones 2007, 771).

ABILITY TO DRAW LINES

Apparently not persuaded of the ability of humans to draw lines, Eric Cohen holds a bleak view of unchecked reproduction:

> Such novel degradations—some imminent, some projects—include the production of cloned children, the creation of children with two male or two female genetic parents, the creation of children with dead embryos or

dead fetuses as parents, the implantation of human embryos into animal wombs, the creation of hybrid embryos using animal sperm and human eggs (or vice versa), and growing parental control over the genetic characteristics of offspring. At stake is not only the dignity of nascent human life, but what it means to be a parent and child, a mother and father, and even what it means to be a human being. (Cohen 2005, 3)

In 1971, Kass wrote that "production of man-animal chimeras by the introduction of selected nonhuman material into developing human embryos is also expected. Fusion of human and nonhuman cells in tissue culture has already been achieved" (Kass 1971, 781). Later, he repeated this and added that the "scientific grapevine also reports attempts (thus far unsuccessful), using artificial fertilization, to cross human egg or sperm with sperm or egg of other primates" (Kass 1985, 22). He wrote this about chimeras: "Finally, the generation of man-animal hybrids or chimeras has been predicted by some reputable scientists. These might be produced by the introduction of selected nonhuman genetic material into the developing human embryos. Fusion of human and nonhuman cells in tissue culture has already been achieved, and so has the transfer of functional genes, from one species into another, by means of the new techniques of DNA recombination" (Kass 1985, 50).

From this perspective, ISR is one of the "distinct threats" posed by biotechnology. It threatens the "degradation of human procreation and the human family, by turning pregnancy into a research technique, by transgressing the species boundary between human and non-human life" (Cohen 2005, 3). What its advocates call conservative bioethics rejects cloning, genetic engineering, and research that would "blur the line between human and nonhuman procreation by seeking to produce humans with animal traits or animals with human traits" (Cohen 2006, 50). The Ethics and Public Policy Center recommends limits on reproduction-related biotechnology and on innovative ways of making babies and experiments that blur the line between humans and other species. The latter would include "the implantation of a human embryo into a nonhuman uterus, or the fusion of animal sperm and human egg or human sperm and animal egg in the effort to produce a hybrid embryo" (Cohen 2006, 53).

Interspecies work, writes Yuval Levin, is a taboo, or a "deep violation or corruption" that would involve the "transgressing of a boundary, or a mixing together of things that ought to be kept separate" (Levin 2003, 54). Eric Cohen commended the 2004 President's Council on Bioethics (PCB) report on reproduction in which "the Council sought to erect barriers that would keep human procreation human: barriers against crossing the boundary between the human and the non-human" (Cohen 2005, 4).

Skeptics may be persuaded that once certain technologies start, it is difficult if not impossible to apply brakes to the momentum. The slippery slope mindset advises not starting in the first place. C. S. Lewis, who had been influenced by *Brave New World* and the eugenics policies under the totalitarian regime in Germany, saw biotechnology as fearful. He wrote in his 1944 book, *The Abolition of Man*, of a "final stage" in which "Man by eugenics, by pre-natal conditioning, and by an education and propaganda based on a perfect applied psychology, has obtained full control over himself," only this mastery is illusory (Lewis 1996, 69). In fact, technology gives power to the few. Just when it seems that humans have conquered nature, it turns out that "the whole human race [is] subjected to some individual men, and those individuals subjected to that in themselves which is purely 'natural'—to their irrational impulses." To Lewis, "Man's conquest of Nature turns out, in the moment of its consummation, to be Nature's conquest of Man."

Three decades later Kass echoed these sentiments when he wrote that "biotechnology is qualitatively different from other technologies because "man can for the first time recreate himself" (Kass 1971, 779). Quoting Lewis he wrote: "Each new power won *by* man is a power *over* man as well" (Kass 1971, 782). Skeptical that humans can control biotechnology, he wrote "the burgeoning technological powers to intervene in the human body and mind, justly celebrated for their contributions to human welfare, are also available for uses that could slide us down the dehumanizing path toward what C. S. Lewis called, in a powerful little book by that name, the abolition of man" (Kass 2002, 3). It is not humans in general who achieve power, but it is some people over others (Kass 1971, 782). Mary Midgley wrote warily of the "hype, the scale of the proposed project, the weight of the economic forces now backing it, and the sweeping change of attitude that is being demanded" of biotechnology (Midgley 2000, 8). There is, as she saw it, an uncritical energy of biotechnological development, a "huge uncriticized impetus, this indiscriminate, infectious corporate overconfidence, this obsessive one-way channeling of energy" (Midgley 2000, 12).

This skepticism also reflects an element of distrust of scientists and the scientific enterprise and of their ability to halt what they have set in motion. Concern about "mischief done by 'rogues'" voiced in discussions within the PCB reappeared in President Bush's remark about "egregious science" and "animal-human hybrids" in his State of the Union message (President's Council on Bioethics 2004, 220; State of the Union 2006). One member pondered why it would be wrong to create a humanzee. "What is offensive here is the mastery," he said, "and this is the ultimate in mastery" (President's Council on Bioethics 2003b, 5). Midgley suggests that "mixed monsters," such as minotaurs and gorgons, "stand for a deep and threatening disorder, something not just confusing but dreadful and invasive" (Midgley 2000, 10).

On the ideologically polar position "transhumanism" stands as a champion of unfettered development of technology. Transhumanists promote research to change the human evolutionary course. Believers in a technological utopia—Rodney Brooks, Hans P. Moravec, Ray Kurzweil, and others—support efforts to enhance human functions so dramatically that humans would enter a state of being "posthuman" (Transhumanism n.d., 1). Humans have an ethical obligation to improve human life according to this view, and they can reach a stage beyond Darwin wherein humans will control their own evolution and "natural evolution would be replaced with deliberate change" (4). Here "natural" is something to be overcome, not protected.

Transhumanists support biotechnology, along with nanotechnology, information technology, and cognitive science, and they believe "nonhuman and part-human animals" should be part of ethical consideration (McKibben 2003, 4, 6). Some envision a nonbiological future led by nanotechnology and other applications. Kurzweil calls this the "singularity" (Kurzweil 2005, 2). He predicts that biotechnology will eventually fade out, and human biology will change through nanotechnology and nanobots (molecular robots). "By the 2040s," he writes, "nonbiological intelligence will be billions of times more capable than our biological intelligence. . . . We are becoming cyborgs" (Kurzweil 2005, 309).

Fears of unstoppable biotechnology have a history. The news of r-DNA technology in the 1970s created a buzz, as illustrated by political cartoons that brought animation and imagination to the microorganisms. In one cartoon a man in a three-piece suit runs down a city street, arms pumping and calling out, "Run for the hills—the recombinant DNA has escaped!" In another, amoeba-like blobs sit on New York City stoops with hats on their heads as an urbane couple walks by and comments, "Remember when there was all that fuss about recombinant DNA?" All conveyed a message of uncontrolled recombined organisms.

The history of genetically modified organisms reveals a more controlled unfolding of transgenics, however, in which oversight and public planning play an important part. This includes the meeting of biologists at Asilomar in 1974, the development of containment guidelines for genetically modified organisms, the initiation of heightened scrutiny for somatic cell gene transfer studies, and the establishment of the Recombinant DNA Advisory Committee. With the prospects of mapping and sequencing the human genome, the U.S. Government set aside funds to study the ethical, legal, and social implications of the Human Genome Project. More recently policy groups convened to examine early ISR, which suggests something other than a downward slope. It is true that in a capitalist society one can expect a momentum to invent, discover, produce, and market. But continued expansion is met with stops along the way for policy adjustments that affect the direction and pace of expansion.

These visions—the conservative's view of a slope down and the transhumanist's view of a streamlined elevator up—are on the edges of contemporary thinking. Alex Mauron and Jean-Marie Thevoz described issues in bioethics in general, whereby "the slippery slope really looks more like a ramshackle staircase: once in a while, we trip down a few steps. This makes us wake up, take stock of ethical shortcomings, and climb up the stairs by appropriate measures such as societal regulation" (Mauron and Thevoz 1991, 658).

DIFFERENCES BETWEEN HUMANS AND NONHUMANS

Julian Savulescu is unusual in seeing potential good in genetic interchange between early-stage humans and nonhumans. As long as the intent is not to create beings for exploitation and is instead to promote human health, such research should not be limited. He argues: "Bringing animals closer to human beings to share their genes might paradoxically improve our humanity . . . . Now we are entering a new phase of human evolution—evolution under reason—where human beings are masters of their destiny. . . . Actions that express or promote rationality are expressions of our humanity" (Savulescu 2003, 24).

The distinction between human and nonhuman animals permeates attitudes toward interspecies studies and goes a long way in explaining why some interspecies studies are deemed threatening. At root the concept of species is fairly straightforward. A species is situated at the base of a classification system for organizing animals and other organisms that subdivides from Kingdom to Phylum, Class, Order, Family, Genus, and Species. Approximately 1.75 million species (including all living organisms) have been described in the world today, and many more remain to be discovered. Of the known species around 5500 are mammalian. At the same time, many other species are in the process of becoming or have already become extinct. Among predecessor human species that became extinct are *Homo neanderthalensis, Homo erectus, Homo habilis,* and *Homo ergaster* (Silver 2006, 92).

On the surface a simple organizational tool, the concept of species for biologists has contentious dimensions. According to Ernst Mayr, "There is probably no other concept in biology that has remained as consistently controversial as the species concept" (Mayr 1982, 51). At least twelve serious definitions of species are open for discussion today among biologists, and Darwin himself was skeptical about whether the concept could be defined (Witherly, Perry, and Leja 2001, 6, 10).

One matter is to determine how to categorize individual animals (Ridley 1996; Mayr 1982). This could depend on several variables, including morphology (what the animal looks like), "clusters of variations" (such as long-tailed or short-tailed traits), mating partners (members of a species generally mate only with those of the same species), and shared ancestors (Species n.d., 2). Species boundaries are thought to be indistinct. The idea of impermeable species is a "notoriously unreliable categorical scheme" (Committee on Guidelines 2005, 41). Biologists tend to regard species as a "scientific heuristic device" of organizational utility

(Singleton 2000, 1095–96), and it is a "working model that allows biologists to get on with their work" (Ankeny 2003). Species indicators are "theoretical tools used to generate predictions and further empirical scientific advances" (Karpowicz 2003). According to Donna Haraway a species has a pragmatic use; it is about "defining difference" (Haraway 2003, 15). None of this is enough to "mandate moral significance" (Singleton 2000, 1096).

Ideological differences about the moral status of living organisms also appear in general public debates. In what the Nuffield Council of Bioethics calls the "clear-line view," humans are special, and "all humans possess some morally vital property that all animals lack" (Nuffield Council on Bioethics 2005, xxi). Peter Lawler, for example, regards language as the grounds for a clear line, which means "the difference between a human being and a dolphin is infinitely greater than the difference between a dolphin and an ant" (President's Council on Bioethics 2005c, 13). In contrast, the "moral sliding scale view" places humans at the top and then accepts a graduated moral importance through primates and other mammals. This elevates some animals to a rights-bearing status vis-à-vis humans. Steve Wise uses a series of indicators to determine which animals are sufficiently close to human cognition to deserve higher moral status than other animals; this includes dolphins, primates, and African Gray parrots (Wise 2004).

A third perspective, the "moral equality view," regards humans and nonhumans as morally equal. Peter Singer argues for equal consideration, not necessarily equal treatment, for human and nonhuman animals (Singer 1990, 2). Because even humans have widely different capacities, it would not make sense to require complete equality for animals. He asserts that "equality is a moral idea, not an assertion of fact" (4). The interests of all beings, no matter the sex, race, or human/nonhuman status (5), must be taken into account. Humans thus have an obligation to attend to suffering: "If a being suffers there can be no moral justification for refusing to take that suffering into consideration" (8). Similarly, James Rachels believes "There is no characteristic, or reasonably small set of characteristics, that sets some creatures apart from others as meriting respectful treatment" (Rachels 2004, 169). He continues, "We always have reason not to harm" (Rachels 2004, 170–71).

Drawing a clear line between human and nonhuman animals may reflect religious beliefs such as the belief that humans were created by God and they alone have souls. Renee Mirkes argues that humans are radically different from animals because they have an immaterial as well as material dimension that makes them "discontinuous from all other species" (Mirkes 2006, 113–14). Animals are "totally defined by their materiality" ("the objective world of things, not the subjective world of persons"), but humans are moral and rise above their material dimensions: "In sum, humans differ from all other animals not superficially or by degree, but radically" (113). He writes that humans are different because they are persons, they have self-determination and can rise above instinctual drives, they have dignity and are ends in themselves, they are fundamentally equal, and they have inherent rights "that are theirs by virtue of their being human" (114). According to Thomas Berg it is the human "essence" and the immateriality of the human intellect that are "accounted for by that intrinsically immaterial and formal organizing principle we call the soul" (Berg 2006, 100). Daston and Mitman observe "the Judeo-Christian tradition that humans were the pinnacle of Creation also encouraged claims that humans, being endowed by God with reason and immortal souls, were superior to and qualitatively different from animals" (Daston and Mitman 2005, 4).

Literal readings of the Bible are also used in reaching conclusions that interspecies studies are wrong. The Christian Medical Fellowship of the United Kingdom points out that the biblical account of creation mentions "according to their various kinds" nine times, which indicates to the Fellowship that species lines are not to be breached. Theologian Ted Peters quotes Henry Morris, a creationist who averred that "each system and each organism were created specifically the way God designed them to be, and He intended each to retain its own character" (Peters 2006, 254). Moreover Leviticus 19:19 warns humans not to "mate different kinds of animals" (United Kingdom. Parliament 2007h).

A secular reason for drawing a clear line is to benefit the human species who enjoy the privileged place that stems from it (Robert and Baylis 2003). Noting that species is a construct created by humans, Kimberly Urie et al. argue that species "remains the most stable foundation upon which our anthropocentric and superior human identity rests" (Urie,

Stanley, and Friedman 2003). Because of the perceived bright line between humans and nonhumans, "we afford ourselves all of the arbitrarily manufactured privileges of a dominant group, similar to institutional domination of male gender over female, light skin over dark, rich over poor" a form of "speciesism" (Urie, Stanley, and Friedman 2003). This treats the animal according to his or her group rather than according to his or her traits (Bekoff 2006a, 220). According to Peter Singer, speciesism "is a prejudice or attitude of bias in favor of the interests of one's own species and against those of members of other species" (Singer 1990, 6). It is not clear why membership in a species "should entail radically different moral status" (Bok 2003).

Singer sees a stealthy form of prejudice presuming the moral superiority of humans over all other species that is used, as prejudices are, to favor the dominant group (Singer 2004, 79). Similarly DeGrazia argues that using species to determine moral status is "self-serving for those in whom species prejudice operates strongly" (DeGrazia 2007, 314). To him it makes little sense to use species differences as markers of moral status and to adopt an all-or-nothing tone that asserts humans have full moral status while other nonhuman animals do not (DeGrazia 2007, 316). He concludes that the Great Apes are borderline persons and, in support, he lists studies that show the capacity of these nonhuman primates to engage in, among other things, social manipulation, body self-awareness, social self-awareness, transmission of behaviors from one generation to the next, altruism, and other signs of moral status (321–22).

To be a borderline person is to have full moral status, and, according to DeGrazia, respect given the Great Apes should be equivalent to that accorded humans; namely, they should be used in research only where the participants face no more than minimum risk, where any greater risk is justified by direct benefits to the participants, and where the participants do not show signs of dissent (DeGrazia 2007, 325). Chimeric studies involving transfer of human neurons to primate brains would not meet these standards, as judged by the primates' needs, not by human-centered interests. With research on rodents, too, the animals' needs should be used to evaluate the research, not the dignity interests of humans.

Speciesism can also apply within nonhuman species; giving disproportionate weight to primates, for example, is "chimpocentric" (Bekoff 2006b,

4). It is also discriminatory, Marc Bekoff argues, to refer to "higher" and "lower" species, especially if this justifies lesser treatment of the latter (Bekoff 2006a, 220). Questioning the bright line would require humans to "acknowledge their similarity to nonhumans" and make it impossible to ignore "the pain and suffering human beings have unquestioningly inflicted on nonhumans" (Urie, Stanley, and Friedman 2003).

Darwin himself posited "evolutionary *continuity* among different species," which means behavioral and other differences between humans and nonhumans are "differences of *degree* rather than differences in *kind*" (Bekoff 2006b, 3). This includes emotions and feelings (Bekoff 2006a, 23, 28). To see animals as our kin, writes Midgley, "inevitably leads us in some degree to welcome them, to identify with them, to see their cause as our own," and this is both alluring and frightening (Midgley 2004, 138). Midgley is curious about fearful reactions to the softening of species lines between humans and nonhumans. "The reaction is extremely interesting," she writes. "What is the threat? Articulate apes and cetaceans are scarcely likely to take over the government" (Midgley 2005, 140).

Graduated lines can also be inferred by comparing the genomes of different species, where DNA is shared more often than it is not. With sequencing projects under way for the genomes of over seventy species in late 2006, the study of comparative genomics will allow increasingly refined measurements of the similarities of a wide array of organisms (Constantine 2007). Such studies also reveal more precise bases for differences between human and nonhuman animals. Humans are territorial about their genes, yet it is not a simple matter to lay claim to a "human" gene. As Urie et al. point out, "All of our genes also exist in other animals, as well as in plants, in varying degrees" (Urie, Stanley, and Friedman 2003, n. 1). And Robert and Baylis note: "Indeed, given the evidence that all living things share a common ancestor, there is little (if any) uniquely human DNA" (Robert and Baylis 2003, 4).

According to one developmental biologist, "From a genetic point of view, it's not that animals are higher or lower than we are, it's just that they've adapted differently, and we can study and learn about these adaptations" (Matthew Scott, quoted in Scott 2006, 36). This means human uniqueness cannot be established by genetic referents alone. Instead of a "human" gene, a set of intersecting genes code for traits associated with humans. To refer to "human-source genes" and "nonhuman-source genes" is more accurate than to refer to "human genes" (Glenn 2003).

It is also problematic to say the human genome differs by 0.1 percent from that of the chimpanzee or by a different percentage from another species in that genes program different proteins, so genes between species do not have a pure one-to-one equivalence. It is like saying Harry and Sherry each have a car but Sherry's is more fully loaded than Harry's, with four-wheel drive and heated front seats, whereas Harry's sedan barely makes it through any weather adversity. What matters is the range of things that spring to action after the turn of a key. Gene expression helps explain human intelligence and other attributes because even though two species may have the same gene, that gene may not be expressed in both (Rogers and Kaplan 2004, 180). Thus, "Changes in where, when, and how much a gene is expressed may [instead of proteins encoded by genes] be the real key to [human] uniqueness" (Pennisi 2006, 1909). One set of researchers found ninety-one genes that had changed activity levels since the split between humans and chimps, and "[eighty] of those became more active in the human brain" (Pennisi 2006, 1910). Moreover, gene codes for a protein may be repeated more times in a human than in other animals (Check 2006, 8).

Although 99 percent of the genes in the human and mouse genomes "have direct counterparts in the two species," the genes differ in structure and function and in the way they are regulated (Nuffield Council on Bioethics 2005, 121). The 1 percent that differ can be highly significant. For example, part of the 1 percent difference for mice includes a cluster of genes relating to smell (123). The olfactory abilities of mice and humans presumably are significantly different. The mouse would have trouble sensing predators or finding food without its sophisticated olfactory genes; a human with the same gene cluster, on the other hand, would face challenges living in a highly odiferous world. Reducing genes to numbers downplays the complex interplay of environmental and physiological factors of gene expression.

SUMMARY

Attitudes toward early ISR are linked to various beliefs, including confidence in the ability of humans to draw lines, the wisdom of listening to visceral reactions to scientific scenarios, the goodness of biotechnology, and the unique status of human beings. These beliefs are fundamental; they touch basic outlooks and make biotechnology a political matter with polarities reflecting what might be called conservative and progressive ways of thinking. This in turn makes early ISR a political matter. Messages from two books representing polar views illustrate points of political difference. *Beyond Therapy* is a 2003 report by the President's Council on Bioethics; *Liberation Biology* is a 2005 book by Ronald Bailey, a science journalist (President's Council on Bioethics 2003a; Bailey 2005).

Beyond Therapy questions the reasons biotechnology is pursued in the first place. Not negating the role of biotechnology in meeting legitimate ends geared to addressing health needs, the Council looks at enhancement rather than therapy, defined as the "use of biotechnical power to alter, by direct intervention, not disease processes but the 'normal' workings of the human body and psyche . . . ." (President's Council on Bioethics 2003a, 13). It asks why humans need to improve and enhance themselves: "What exactly is it about the lot of humankind that needs or invites improvement?" It expresses dismay at the seemingly rudderless expansion of biotechnology: "Biotechnology, like any other technology, is not for anything in particular" (3). Whereas bioethics often focuses on the means of developing biotechnology (e.g., by ensuring informed consent), the Council is interested in the ends themselves. What goals are served by biotechnology? Do these goals lead to "human flourishing," or do they lead to "dehumanization" or "superhumanization"? (8). Fearing that humans "will not be satisfied with the average," the Council foresees people striving to improve and enhance in unfulfilling ways that are out of touch with natural human desires and goals (21).

Although early ISR is not explicitly mentioned in this particular volume, other publications of the PCB indicate skepticism of some forms of human-animal change (President's Council on Bioethics 2004). The Council in its volume *Beyond Therapy* does, however, consider and critique the quest for "age retardation" and "life extension," both of which might be achieved with the assistance of early interspecies studies in the quest for regenerative medicine (President's Council on Bioethics 2003a, 164). In this way it would flag not just the animal-human techniques but also the ends toward which the research is aimed. Even basic human-animal interchanges would be suspect if done mindlessly and for enhancement.

Ronald Bailey, on the other hand, defines liberation biology as "the earthly quest to overcome the physical and mental limitations imposed on us by nature, enabling us to flourish as never before" (Bailey 2005, 12). In contrast to the PCB, Bailey believes that enhancement biotechnology aids rather than interferes with human flourishing. Where the PCB looks with dismay at efforts to postpone aging, for example, Bailey holds the opposite view: Because humans have traditionally not lived as long as they do today, "significant aging is a relatively new phenomenon" and is not a natural state (27). Consequently, humans are justified in trying to reverse the effects of aging to maintain the quality of life of a younger human who is in a more natural state (27). Bailey sees the extension of life as "a perfect flourishing of our human nature" (61).

Bailey sees what he calls bioconservatives as engaged in a "political movement to quash biotech development because it conflicts with their notions of human nature" (Bailey 2005, 17). To him these conflicting views involve deliberate efforts to assume and exercise power. He avers that a "new pro-biotech politics must grow to counter the bioconservative ideology of stagnation" (22). Bailey's critique of the precautionary principle illustrates the policy implications of his position. Whereas the PCB would avoid moving into areas where the impact on human happiness was unknown or unexamined, Bailey would not hold back on the basis of speculative concerns. To him a precautionary stance means presuming biotechnologies are "guilty until proven innocent," and with this position, biotechnology would be the loser (242). He argues that the "precautionary principle demands that we restrain technological developments not on the basis of what we know, but on the basis of what we do not know" (244). Noting that predictions about biotechnology can be wrong and that not going ahead will stifle many scientific advances, he calls "wise public policy" that which "allows people, including biomedical researchers, maximum scope to pursue the good and the true in their own ways, in conformity with the dictates of their own consciences" (245). This would include various forms of early ISR when they enable efforts to bring "new opportunities to cure disease, alleviate suffering . . . and lengthen healthy lives" (246).

These synopses highlight some of the political dimensions of early ISR: (1) coherent opposing views about biotech held by individuals who

(2) embrace their position on the conservative or progressive ends of the spectrum and (3) for whom the issue is salient and meaningful. They differ by their (4) readiness to move ahead without full knowledge, (5) conception of what is to be guarded against, and (6) belief in the appropriate ends of the research. Their differences cover not just human-nonhuman techniques but a broader philosophy into which early ISR falls. It is not just a matter of proceeding with technique or not; it is a matter of what kind of world view that technique promotes.

The implication for policy, of course, is that consensus will be elusive. Yet when contrasting views are recognized and mutually respected, the mundane task of policy development can take place if policy modifications are in order. In the United States at least an interchange about the morality of early ISR is taking place alongside a permissive policy context. At present those who do not see early ISR as particularly problematic have held sway, if the dearth of restrictive policies at the national level is a marker. Those who do see ES-cell research as problematic, however, including the members of a number of state legislatures in the United States, have made the climate for ES-cell research, and consequently for early ISR as a methodological adjunct of the research, less inviting.

Conclusion
Is Early Interspecies Research Fundamentally Distinct?

WHAT ARE WE TO MAKE of the place of "animal-human hybrids" in bioethics and policy? Hybrids, along with genetic alterations, cloning, and ectogenesis (artificial uterus), entered the literature of bioethics and policy in the 1970s as a metaphor for unleashed biotechnology. This metaphor continues today: "Some transforming powers are already here. The Pill. In vitro fertilization. Bottled embryos. Surrogate wombs. Cloning. Genetic screening. Genetic manipulation. Organ harvesting. Mechanical spare parts. Chimeras" (Kass 2002, 5). Framed as a future possibility lying at the bottom of a slippery slope, the integration of human and animal biological material for reproductive ends melded into historic visual images of mythical monsters and chimeric oddities. As Turney points out, images such as Frankenstein (his example) or hybrids can elicit a script. "Once a script has been laid down," he writes, "a single cue can evoke an entire story, as an interpretive frame or context for what is being discussed" (Turney 1998, 6).

In recent years with innovative scientific endeavors under way, the script involving the concept of animal-human hybrids has been in transition. Already more detailed policy templates are in the works, with the United Kingdom's integration of "admixed embryos" into its licensing structure a key example. In the United States the fleshing out of guidelines in regenerative medicine institutes in California, New Jersey, and other states provides another venue to develop norms and practices for early interspecies research (ISR). This book challenges the worry-based rudiments of the earlier but largely unexamined script in order to suggest mechanisms for a more empirically based script about the role of early ISR in research on regenerative medicine.

For some types of early ISR more than others, a valley exists between objections and evidence, with the former outpacing the latter. A generous interpretation is that deep-seated values are primarily at issue. A less generous interpretation is that political interests are also at play with exaggerated warnings designed to foment distrust and uncertainty. At root both exist together.

In the United States a line of argument among some objectors is that early ISR will lead to illicit outcomes at the hands of "renegade researchers." This equates chimeric animal-human studies with unseemly science, encompasses a broad sweep with vague reference to animal-human hybrids, and advocates anticipatory bans. It also reflects preexisting divisions related to different views of the moral status of embryos. For example, an antichimera bill introduced in Delaware's legislature specified that a human individual existed "from the beginning of the single-cell stage onward, produced by any means" (Delaware General Assembly 2007). With this stipulation no research would be permissible on human embryos, much less research using human embryos and nonhuman cells together.

Objections to early ISR also surface in academic circles and policy advisory bodies, where the goal is not necessarily to restrict research but instead to flesh out its dimensions in order to ensure it is carried out in an ethically acceptable way. That message is generally one of caution rather than censure.

It should be noted, however, that those in the policy and scientific communities who regard early ISR as legitimate and not particularly troublesome have been relatively quiet in the face of both fanciful and serious objections. For a variety of reasons, reassurances about early ISR from stem-cell supporters are not as crisp as identification of issues by critics. Perhaps those who take early ISR "in stride" (Silver 2006, 187) are not inclined to respond to what they regard as irrational or frivolous objections. Or perhaps they choose not to lend legitimacy to concerns by addressing them, or fail to understand ethical objections, or simply wish not to become involved in what looks like a political imbroglio. Nevertheless when objections are not carefully addressed, an opportunity is missed to examine issues in a way that accepts the role of early ISR in research and development.

With concern about a regulatory "chimaera quagmire" in mind, the editors of the journal *Nature* in 2007 advised readers to take a more active role in "identify[ing] the various research protocols defining interspecies research involving human cells and embryos, and the associated risks, ethical issues and benefits of each" (Avoiding a Chimaera Quagmire 2007). Inasmuch as the journal reaches scientists and policy specialists, this editorial in effect invited diverse voices to help shape the way early ISR is framed in public debate.

If new ways of looking at human-nonhuman studies are in process, it makes sense to investigate individual attitudes about animal-human research, which apparently have been studied by few if any social scientists. A government-sponsored survey in the United Kingdom revealed that respondents were more supportive of research using cybrids if the purpose of the research was explained (Human Fertilisation and Embryology Authority 2007a, Appendix F). Research on the psychological underpinnings of repugnance can also shed light on the bases for intuitive reactions to human-nonhuman research (Jones 2007).

Studies of public attitudes can help explain when human-nonhuman mixes move from acceptable to unacceptable in the minds of critics. If splicing limited human DNA sequences to animals for study is acceptable to critics, why are human-nonhuman chimeras not acceptable? Transgenic animals result from DNA splicing, cybrids from cytoplasm substitution, chimeras from cell mixing, and hybrids from genomic mixing. Current deliberations leave only a vague sense of when the blending is too much and why. Some observers have proposed that anything that causes the creation of beings with both human and nonhuman features or traits is unacceptable, but this is not helpful for contemporary research, which does not lead to observable physiognomic human traits in animals.

Authors who criticize chimeric research because it threatens moral ideas have been criticized for not giving examples of actual ongoing research that is morally confusing (Sagoff 2003). Contemporary studies involve small animals, mild chimerism, and animals that fail to develop or are sacrificed before or shortly after birth. The goal is to further regenerative medicine, not to provoke human features in mice. As Shreeve asks, "Does even the fleeting, prenatal existence of a chimera of unknown aspect cross a moral line—not because of what it might look like or become but simply for what it is?" (Shreeve 2005, 45).

For all the attention given to animal-human hybrids, there is little or no interest in fertilizing human and animal gametes for research. A key difference between research and application exists for all these techniques; creating a microscopic interspecies entity and destroying it within days is a separate matter from transferring that entity to the uterus of an animal or human for development and birth. As one group of stem-cell researchers put it, the images of chimeras and hybrids "imply a living creature with features that are both human and animal, and this is grossly misleading when compared to the reality of what is being proposed" (United Kingdom. Parliament 2007e). As an investigator said of cybrids, "you have to understand that we are using very, very little information from the cow in order to do this reprogramming idea" (BBC News 2007).

If ethical objections to date lack significant ballast, it is difficult to form a rationale for restrictive regulation. Policymaking includes taking no action, integrating oversight into existing frameworks, and crafting new laws with early ISR in mind. To what extent, if any, does early ISR raise sufficiently distinct issues to require policy adjustments? The chapters above indicate that policy problems are not so great as to require new laws. Instead, a course of watchful deliberation can suffice, or modifications can be made to existing frameworks. These frameworks take different forms across political systems. Interspecies research can be integrated into licensing systems in the United Kingdon and Canada, for example, and into voluntary guidelines for human embryos or ES-cell research in the United States. Countries vary in their approaches to other areas of medicine, including assisted reproductive technologies (ARTs). A survey in 1998 revealed that twenty of thirty-eight nations oriented their ART policy around a legislative approach, whereas eleven used guidelines from professional societies, and seven had neither legislation nor guidelines (Jones and Cohen 1999, 7).

The preceding chapters suggest that no compelling reason exists at present to regard early ISR as fundamentally distinct. Rather, the ends (or products) matter more than the particular techniques (or process). Flagging research because animal cells are present is a process-based approach, similar to flagging crops that have been genetically modified by recombinant-DNA techniques. In both cases it is the technique (process) that attracts policy attention in the first place and presumes heightened oversight. This book was organized by technique (process) in that it highlighted studies by the mutual presence of human and nonhuman cells, tissues, or genes. Yet it concludes that this mixed presence does not in itself signal harms serious enough for heightened review. Instead a preferable approach might be a product-based focus on research outcomes.

One can ask, however, if anything would be wrong with a national government passing a comprehensive law that bars licenses for variations of early ISR, such as the licensing systems in the United Kingdom or Canada. Arguably this could promote public acceptance of investigations, as in the United Kingdom's experience with cybrids. It could also add to the armamentarium of principles and guidelines for countries without detailed policies. On the other hand, it could prematurely cut off debate about the research in question through inflexible restrictions. If broadly written, restrictions can foreclose more research than intended or needed. Moreover, in the absence of solid justifications, such laws can perpetuate misinformation and fail to accommodate changes in values over time. As Green states, "Almost no prohibition can be absolute in a world in which today's imaginative possibility is tomorrow's widely demanded clinical procedure" (Green 2001, 97).

Anticipatory restraints can also discourage a careful explication of values. David Guston writes that "policies are, and should rightly be, about articulating public values" (Guston 2008, 940). An oversight system is more nuanced than a stand-alone ban, which shuts down discussion. Ted Peters wrote that "to label all this 'chimerism' and then forbid it categorically would be tantamount to cutting off the electricity and water supply to the laboratory and the hospital." As an alternative he offered that "precaution, not prohibition, is the road reason ought to take through the wilderness of moral confusion" (Peters 2006, 257–58).

At root, the form of oversight depends on a country's policy context. Yet no matter what the location, technological imminence and evidence of risks and benefits are needed for informed policy to be crafted. Without immediacy, the danger rises of speculation, emotion-based conclusions, and conceptual confusion. Research need not be forbidden altogether; in the United States, where no explicit national framework covers research involving human embryos, an alternative is to incorporate early ISR into existing ES-cell guidelines, as was done by the Committee on Guidelines, CIRM, and ISSCR.

Early ISR presents the opportunity to think and act in ways that recognize the interests of both humans and nonhumans. In the United States agencies with authority over animal biotechnology and with distinct statutory mandates include the Animal and Plant Health Inspection Service (APHIS), Office of Laboratory Animal Welfare (NIH), Center for Veterinary Medicine of FDA, and Center for Drug Evaluation and Research of FDA. Although these agencies lack a central regulatory framework specifying who is responsible, their policies accord protections to animals used in research (National Research Council 2002, 113, 162).

In addition early ISR can advance awareness of prejudicial ways of thinking about animals in research. The current paradigm, writes Midgley, includes a tendency to talk about humans and then dismiss "animals" as an unrefined enormous generic whole when, in fact, the animal kingdom is tremendously complex, with creatures ranging from "blue whales to tiny micro-organisms" (Midgley 2004, 135). At issue is more than rules. At issue is "widening of the circle of human empathy and sympathy" to include animals (Daston and Mitman 2005, 5) and to ask "how can we preserve human rights and human dignity despite the fact that our 'humanness' might no longer be the exclusive possession of *Homo sapiens*?" (Glenn 2003).

David Favre has dryly observed that the "U.S. President is hardly likely to declare that 'It is time that we do something for the animals'" (Favre 2004, 90, 92). The absence of leadership at the top leaves it to others in the policy community to strengthen norms that protect animals in research and to follow the recommendations of the three-*R* approach. It also opens the door to appreciating the complexity of nonhuman animals with reference to the growing body of knowledge about animal cognition and personality (e.g., Wise 2002; Nussbaum 2004; Sunstein and Nussbaum 2004; Bekoff 2006b).

The matter of early ISR is a study in societal responses to what could easily become sensationalized science. The policies in the United States reveal caution in rule making and little if any official reaction to early ISR.

It is clear that policies enacted years ago in a number of countries bar certain forms of animal-human research. It remains to be seen whether recent laws also crimp research. In the United Kingdom, for example, regulations governing the use of cybrids have promoted rather than diminished inquiry.

For all the displays of images of Greek chimeras over time, the contemporary response to real chimeras has been confused but understated. In some ways it can serve as a template for shifts of focus in future years to nonbiological and mechanistic therapies and a new set of images: cyborgs, Blade Runner, synthetic biology, genomic design, and artificial chromosomes come to mind. Julian Savulescu notes that people may find the "introduction of animal genetic material into human beings more repugnant and bestial than the introduction of nonbiological material" but that the "scope for radical differences in artificial life" is much greater than the scope for animals, which are limited by "the range of genes that occur naturally" (Savulescu 2003, 25). Viewed as a step toward technologies yet to come, the study of early ISR demonstrates how the search for a common conceptual language, patience in fleshing out issues, and a willingness to forgo sensational imagery all contribute to reasoned policies. If the hyperbolic side of early ISR has failed to translate to fear-based legislation at the national level, this is in part because of our willingness to deliberate with curiosity.

References

Abbott, Alison. 1999. Three *Rs* could make laboratories a better place for animals. *Nature* 401:106.

———. 2004. Geneticists prepare for deluge of mutant mice. *Nature* 432:541.

Ainsworth, Claire. 2003. The stranger within. *New Scientist* 180 (2421): 34.

Allhoff, Fritz. 2005. Germ-line enhancement and Rawlsian primary goods. *Kennedy Institute of Ethics Journal* 15 (1): 39–56.

Alper, Joe. 2003. Hatching the golden egg: a new way to make drugs. *Science* 300:729–30.

Andrews, Lori B. n.d. How art challenges us to consider the human future. Institute on Biotechnology and the Human Future. Chicago-Kent College of Law; Illinois Institute of Technology. Available at www.thehumanfuture.org/themes/arts/. Accessed April 16, 2009.

Animal Testing. 2006. Available at http://en.wikipedia.org/wiki/Animal_testing. Accessed November 3, 2006.

Ankeny, Rachel A. 2003. No real categories, only chimeras and illusions: the interplay between morality and science in debates over embryonic chimeras. *American Journal of Bioethics* 3 (3): 31–33.

Anker, Suzanne, and Dorothy Nelkin. 2004. *The Molecular Gaze: Art in the Genetic Age.* Cold Spring Harbor, NY: Cold Spring Harbor Laboratory Press.

ARC Centre for Kangaroo Genomics. n.d. Artificial reproduction strategies to achieve hybridisation. Available at http://kangaroo.genomics.org.au. Accessed April 23, 2007.

Asia. n.d. Available at http://www.glphr.org/genetic/asia2-07.htm. Accessed October 20, 2005.

Assay for Sperm Quality. US Patent 6103481. Issued on August 15, 2000. Available at http://www.patentstorm.us/patents/6103481-description.html Accessed February 5, 2007.

Association of American Medical Colleges. 2005. Human Embryonic Stem Cell Research: Regulatory and Administrative Challenges. The Report of an AAMC Workshop by Katharina Phillips, Susan Ehringhaus, and Anthony Mazzaschi. Available at www.amc.org. Accessed June 18, 2007.

Australia Approves Use of Cloned Human Embryos. 2006. *New Scientist.* November 8. Available at www.newscientist.com/article/dn10469-australia. Accessed on August 3, 2008.

Austriaco, Nicanor Pier Giorgio. 2006. How to navigate species boundaries: a reply to *The American Journal of Bioethics. National Catholic Bioethics Quarterly* 6 (1): 61–71.

Avoiding a chimaera quagmire. 2007. *Nature* 445:1.

Bailey, Ronald. 2005. *Liberation Biology: The Scientific and Moral Case for the Biotech Revolution.* Amherst, NY: Prometheus Books.

Baker, Monya. 2009. Fast and furious. *Nature* 458:962–65.

Balkenhol, Stephan. 1995. Three Hybrids, 1995. Shown at the Hirshhorn Museum and Sculpture Garden. Available at http://hirshhorn.si.edu/visit/collection_object.asp?key=32&subkey=2844. Accessed June 22, 2006.

Baylis, Françoise. 2008. Animal eggs for stem cell research: a path not worth taking. *American Journal of Bioethics* 8 (12): 18–32.

Baylis, Françoise, and Jason Scott Robert. 2007. Part-human chimeras: worrying the facts, probing the ethics. *American Journal of Bioethics* 7 (5): 41–58.

Baylis, Françoise, and Andrew Fenton. 2007. Chimera research and stem cell therapies for human neurodegenerative disorders. *Cambridge Quarterly of Healthcare Ethics* 16:195–208.

Bazopoulou-Kyrkanidou, Euterpe. 2001. Chimeric creatures in Greek mythology and reflections in science. *American Journal of Medical Genetics* 100:66–80.

BBC News. 2007. Human-animal embryo green light. September 5. Available at http://news.bbc.co.uk/1/ni/health/6978384.stm. Accessed June 3, 2008.

Bekoff, Marc. 2006a. Emotions, cognition, and animal selves: "Wow! That's me!" In *Animal Passions and Beastly Virtues: Reflections on Redecorating Nature,* edited by Marc Bekoff, 23–34. Philadelphia: Temple University Press.

———. 2006b. Ethics, compassion, conservation, and activism: redecorating nature. In *Animal Passions and Beastly Virtues: Reflections on Redecorating Nature,* edited by Marc Bekoff, 219–24. Philadelphia: Temple University Press.

Berg, Thomas. 2006. Human brain cells in animal brains: philosophical and moral considerations. *National Catholic Bioethics Quarterly* 6 (1): 89–107.

Biologists weigh up risks of synthetic genomes. 2005. *Nature* 435:1151.

Board on Life Sciences (The National Academies) and Board on Health Sciences Policy (Institute of Medicine). 2004. Interspecies mixing and chimeras.

Session at Public Workshop sponsored by Guidelines for Human Embryonic Stem Cell Research. October 12–13, 2004, Washington, DC. PowerPoint and presentation notes available at http://dels.nas.edu/bls/stemcells/powerpoints .html. Accessed on March 1, 2007; site now discontinued.

Bok, Hilary. 2003. What's wrong with confusion? *American Journal of Bioethics* 3 (3): 25–26.

Bonnicksen, Andrea L. 2002. *Crafting a Cloning Policy: From Dolly to Stem Cells.* Washington, DC: Georgetown University Press.

Boyd Group. 1999. Genetic Engineering: Animal Welfare and Ethics: A discussion paper from the Boyd Group. September 1999. Available at www.boyd-group .demon.co.uk/genmod.htm. Accessed December 26, 2006.

Braga, Daniela Paes de Almedia Ferreira, Fabio Firmbach Pasqualatto, Camila Madaschi, et al. 2007. Use of pig oocytes for training new professionals in human assisted reproduction laboratories. *Fertility and Sterility* 88 (5): 1408–12.

Buchanan, Allen, Dan W. Brock, Norman Daniels, and Daniel Winkler. 2000. *From Chance to Choice: Genetics and Justice.* Cambridge, UK: Cambridge University Press.

BVAAWF/FRAME/RSPCA/UJFAW Joint Working Group on Refinement. 2003. Refinement and reduction in production of genetically modified mice. Sixth report. Available at www.lal.org.uk/pdffiles/transgenic.pdf. Accessed November 3, 2006 .

California Institute for Regenerative Medicine. 2007. CIRM MES Regulations Title 17 California Code of Regulations Section 100010-100110. CIRM Revised January 31, 2007.

Canada/Government. 2004. An Act Respecting Human Reproduction and Related Research. Bill C-6. Ottawa. 29 March. Available at http://laws.justice .gc.ca/en/a-13.4/218740.html Accessed June 20, 2006.

Canadian Institutes of Health Research. 2006. Updated Guidelines for Human Pluripotent Stem Cell Research (June 28). Available at www.irsc.gc.ca/e/31488 .html. Accessed August 1, 2008.

Castle, David. 2003. Hopes against hopeful monsters. *American Journal of Bioethics* 3 (3): 28–29.

Caulfield, Timothy, and Roger Brownsword. 2006. Human dignity: a guide to policy making in the biotechnology era? *Nature Reviews Genetics* 7:72–76.

Center for American Progress. 2006. Bioethics and politics: past, present, and future. Panel I. The emergence of politicized bioethics. Transcript. April 21, 2006. Available at www.americanprogress.org. Accessed July 5, 2006.

Centre for Stem Cell Biology and Developmental Genetics. Institute of Human Genetics. University of Newcastle upon Tyne. n.d. Derivation of embryonic stem cell lines from interspecies embryos produced by somatic cell nuclear transfer (R0179). Research application to HFEA (summary). Available at http://www.hfea.gov.uk/en/1652.html. Accessed February 27, 2008.

Chapman, Audrey R., and Mark S. Frankel, eds. 2003. *Designing our Descendants: The Promises and Perils of Genetic Modifications.* Baltimore: Johns Hopkins University Press.

Charo, R. Alta. 2004. Passing on the right: conservative bioethics is closer than it appears. *Journal of Law, Medicine & Ethics* 32 (2): 307–14.

Check, Erika. 2006. Mix and match: the hunt for what makes us human. *Nature* 443:8–9.

Cheshire, William P. 2007. The moral musings of a murine chimera. *American Journal of Bioethics* 7 (5): 49–50.

Chimera [genetics]. n.d. http://en.wikipedia.org/wiki/Chimera_(genetics). Accessed July 25, 2006.

Chimera on a bike? 2005. *Science* 308:1864.

Chong, Dennis, and James N. Druckman. 2007. Framing theory. *Annual Review of Political Science* 10:103–26.

Clinical Sciences Research Institute, University of Warwick. n.d. The generation of human embryonic stem cells by transferring a human cell into recipient pig eggs. Research application to HFEA (summary). Available at http://www.hfea.gov.uk/en/375.html. Accessed February 27, 2008.

Clinton, William J. 1998. Letter to Harold Shapiro of NBAC on November 14, 1998. Washington, DC: The White House.

Cobbe, Neville. 2007. Cross-species chimeras: exploring a possible Christian perspective. *Zygon* 42 (3): 599–622.

Cohen, Cynthia. 2007a. Beyond the human neural mouse to the NAS guidelines. *American Journal of Bioethics* 7 (5): 46–49.

———. 2007b. *Renewing the Stuff of Life: Stem Cells, Ethics, and Public Policy.* New York: Oxford University Press.

Cohen, Eric. 2005. The bioethics agenda and the Bush second term. *The New Atlantis* 7 (Fall 2004/Winter 2005): 1–6.

———. 2006. Conservative bioethics and the search for wisdom. *Hastings Center Report* 36 (1): 44–56.

Colorado State University. n.d. Mosaicism and chimerism. Available at http://arbl.cvmbs.colostate.edu/hbooks/genetics/medgen/chromo/mosaics.html. Accessed July 25, 2006.

Committee on Guidelines for Human Embryonic Stem Cell Research, National Research Council, Institute of Medicine. 2005. *Guidelines for Human Embryonic Stem Cell Research.* Washington, DC: National Academies Press.

Constantine, David. 2007. Close-ups of the genome, species by species by species. *New York Times,* January 23, D4.

Cosmides, Leda, and John Tooby. n.d. Evolutionary psychology: a primer. Available at http://www.psych.ucsb.edu/research/cep/primer.html. Accessed January 11, 2008.

Council of Europe. Parliamentary Assembly. 1986. "Recommendation 1046 (1986) on the use of human embryos and foetuses for diagnostic, therapeutic, scientific, industrial and commercial purposes." Available at http://assembly.coe .int/Maineasp?Link=http%3A//assembly.coe.int/Documents/AdoptedText/ ta86/EREC1046.htm. Accessed January 16, 2009.

Crichton, Michael. 2006. *Next.* New York: HarperCollins Publishers.

Cyranoski, David. 2007. Simple switch turns cells embryonic. *Nature* 447:618–19.

Daston, Lorraine, and Gregg Mitman. 2005. The how and why of thinking with animals. In *Thinking with Animals: New Perspectives on Anthropomorphism,* edited by Lorraine Daston and Gregg Mitman, 1–14. New York: Columbia University Press.

Davis v. Davis 842 S.W. 2d 588 (Tenn. 1992).

Dawkins, Richard. 2009. Richard Dawkins: how would you feel about a half-human half-chimp hybrid? Available at www.guardian.co.uk/science/blog/2009/ Jan/02/richard-dawkins-chimpanzee-hybrid. Accessed January 8, 2009.

Daylon, James, Scott N. Noggle, Tomasz Swigut, et al. 2006. Contribution of human embryonic stem cells to mouse blastocysts. *Developmental Biology* 295 (1): 90–102.

DeGrazia, David. 2007 Human-animal chimeras: human dignity, moral status, and species prejudice. *Metaphilosophy* 38 (2–3): 309–29.

Delaware General Assembly. 2007. An Act to Prohibit Human and Human/ Non-Human Cloning in Delaware. H.B. 76. House of Representatives. 144th General Assembly. Available at http://www.legis.delaware.gov/LIS/LIS144.NSF/ 93487d394bc01014882569a4007a4cb7/b74153538f19141985257275004c22bc ?OpenDocument. Accessed November 1, 2008.

Denmark. 1988. Law No. 353 of 3 June 1987 on the Establishment of an Ethical Council and the Regulation of Certain Forms of Biomedical Research. Lovtidende for Kongeriget Danmark. Part A, 3 June 1987. No. 44. Reprinted in *International Digest of Health Legislation* 39 (1): 95–97.

Dennis, Carina. 2006. Off by a whisker. *Nature* 442:739–41.

Derbes, V. J. 1966. De Mussis and the Great Plague of 1348: a forgotten episode of bacteriological warfare. *JAMA* 196:179–82.

Dewan, Shaila. 2009. After change in federal policy, some states take steps to limit stem cell research. *New York Times.* March 14, p. A8.

DeWitt, Natalie. 2002. Biologists divided over proposal to create human-mouse embryos. *Nature* 420:255.

ECVAM Workshop 28. n.d. The use of transgenic animals in the European Union: the report and recommendations of ECVAM Workshop 28. Available at http://altweb.jhsph.edu/publications/ecvam/ecvam28.htm. Accessed November 8, 2006.

Edelman, Murray. 1995. *From Art to Politics: How Artistic Creations Shape Political Conceptions.* Chicago: University of Chicago Press.

Elias, Paul. 2006. Mixing animal and human cells gets more exotic. Available at http://www.mercurynews.com/mld/mercurynews/news/local/states/california. Accessed June 19, 2006.

Endy, Drew. 2005. Foundations for engineering biology. *Nature* 438:449–53.

ESHRE Task Force on Ethics and Law. 2001. I. The moral status of the pre-implantation embryo. *Human Reproduction* 16 (5): 1046–48.

Ethics Advisory Board, Department of Health, Education, and Welfare. 1979. *Appendix: HEW Support of Research Involving Human In Vitro Fertilization and Embryo Transfer.* Washington, DC: Government Printing Office, May 4.

Ethics Committee of the American Fertility Society. 1986. Ethical considerations of the new reproductive technologies. *Fertility and Sterility* 46:1S–94S.

Ethics Committee of the American Society for Reproductive Medicine. 1997. Informed consent and the use of gametes and embryos for research. *Fertility and Sterility* 68:780–81.

———. 2002. Donating spare embryos for embryonic stem-cell research. *Fertility and Sterility* 78:957–60.

Favre, David. 2004. Integrating animal interests into our legal system. *Animal Law* 10:87–97.

Fehilly, C. B., S. M. Willadsen, and E. M. Tucker. 1984. Interspecies chimaerism between sheep and goat. *Nature* 307:634–36.

Frankel, Mark S., and Audrey R. Chapman. 2000. *Human Inheritable Genetic Modifications: Assessing Scientific, Ethical, Religious, and Policy Issues.* Washington, DC: American Association for the Advancement of Science.

Friends of Washoe. n.d. Available at www.friendsofwashoe.org. Accessed September 14, 2008.

Fukuyama, Francis, and Franco Furger. 2006. *Beyond Bioethics: A Proposal for Modernizing the Regulation of Human Biotechnologies.* Washington, DC: Paul H. Nitze School of Advanced International Studies.

Gardner, R. L. 1968. Mouse chimeras obtained by the injection of cells into the blastocyst. *Nature* 220:596–97.

Geep. n.d. www.greenapple.com/~jorp/amzanim/cross08a.htm. Accessed August 18, 2006; site now discontinued.

Gelada Baboon (*Theropithecus gelada*). 2006. Available at http://www.theprimata .com/theropithecus_gelada.html. Accessed November 8, 2006.

Genetic Mosaics. n.d. Available at http://users.rcn.com/jkimball.ma.ultranet/ biology/m/mosaics.html#tetragametichuman. Accessed September 18, 2006; site now discontinued.

Genetics and Public Policy Center. 2005. *Human Germline Genetic Modification: Issues and Options for Policymakers.* Washington, DC: Genetics and Public Policy Center.

Geron Ethics Advisory Board. 1999. Research with human embryonic stem cells: ethical considerations. *Hastings Center Report* 29 (2): 31–36.

Glenn, Linda MacDonald. 2003. A legal perspective on humanity, personhood, and species boundaries. *American Journal of Bioethics* 3 (3): 27–28.

Greely, Henry T. 2003. Defining Chimeras . . . and Chimeric Concerns. *American Journal of Bioethics* 3 (3): 17–20.

Greely, Henry T., Mildred K. Cho, Linda F. Hogle, and Debra M. Satz. 2007. Thinking about the human neuron mouse. *American Journal of Bioethics* 7 (5): 27–40.

Green, Ronald M. 2001. *The Human Embryo Research Debates: Bioethics in the Vortex of Controversy.* New York: Oxford University Press.

Greene, Mark, Kathryn Schill, Shoji Takahashi, et al. 2005. Moral issues of human- non-human primate neural grafting. *Science* 309:385–86.

Grimm, David G. 2006. A mouse for every gene. *Science* 312:1862–66.

Guston, David H. 2008. Innovation policy: not just a jumbo shrimp. *Nature* 454:940–41.

Hall, Stephen S. 2006. Stem cells: a status report. *Hastings Center Report* 36 (1): 16–22.

Halme, Dina Gould, and David A. Kessler. 2006. FDA regulation of stem-cell- based therapies. *New England Journal of Medicine* 355 (16): 1730–35.

Hanna, Kathi E. 2007. Ball of confusion: how stem cells have stymied review boards. *Thomson Center Watch* 4:128–36.

Haraway, Donna. 2003. *The Companion Species Manifesto: Dogs, People, and Significant Otherness.* Chicago: Prickly Paradigm Press, 2003.

Harris, John. 2007. *Enhancing Evolution: The Ethical Case for Making Better People.* Princeton: Princeton University Press.

Hayden, Erika Check, and Monya Baker. 2009. Virus-free pluripotency for human cells. *Nature* 458:19.

Henderson, Mark, and Francis Elliott. 2008. MPs back creation of human-animal embryos. *The Times,* May 20. Available at http://www.timesonline.co.uk/tol/news/politics/article3964693.ece. Accessed July 22, 2008.

Hinxton Group. 2008. Asia and Oceania: Policy Excerpts. Available at www.hinxtongroup.org/wp_ao_exc.html. Accessed November 11, 2008.

Ho, Mae-Wan. 2000. *Genetic Engineering: Dream or Nightmare?* 2nd ed. New York: Continuum Publishing Company.

Holden, Constance, and Gretchen Vogel. 2004. A technical fix for an ethical bind? *Science* 306:2174–76.

Human Fertilisation and Embryology Authority. 2007a. Hybrids and Chimeras: A Report on the Findings of the Consultation. October. Available at http://www.hfea.gov.uk/docs/Hybrids_Report.pdf. Accessed June 28, 2007.

———. 2007b. Research News. Use of Animal Eggs in Embryo Research. Available at http://www.hfea.gov.uk/en/377.html. Accessed February 2, 2007.

Human Genetics Advisory Committee. 1998. Cloning issues in reproduction, science and medicine. Available at http://www.advisorybodies.doh.gov.uk/hgac/papers/papers_c.htm. Accessed March 3, 2006.

Humanzee. n.d. Available at http://en.wikipedia.org/wiki/Humanzee. Accessed August 18, 2006.

International Stem Cell Forum Ethics Working Party. 2006. Ethics issues in stem cell research. *Science* 312:366–67.

Interstate Alliance on Stem Cell Research. 2008. Agenda: September 9–10, 2008. Available at www.iascr.org/docs/agenda-sep2008.pdf. Accessed December 20, 2008.

ISSCR. 2006. Guidelines for the Conduct of Human Embryonic Cell Research, Version 1: December 21, 2006. Available at www.isscr.org/guidelines/index.htm. Accessed February 12, 2007.

Items of Interest about Hybrids. n.d. Available at www.greenapple.com/~jorp/amzanim/interest.htm. Accessed August 18, 2006.

Johnston, Josephine, and Christopher Eliot. 2003. Chimeras and human dignity. *American Journal of Bioethics* 3 (3): 6–7.

Jolly, Clifford J., Tamsin Woolley-Barker, Shimelis Beyene, Todd R. Disotell, and Jane E. Phillips-Conroy. 1997. Intergenetic hybrid baboons. *International Journal of Primatology* 18 (4): 597–627.

Jones, Dan. 2007. The depths of disgust. *Nature* 447:768–71.

Jones, Howard W. Jr., and Jean Cohen. 1999. Surveillance 1998. Available at www.mnet.fr/iffs/a_surv.htm. Accessed April 3, 2001; site now discontinued.

Juengst, Eric T. 1991. Germ-line gene therapy: back to basics. *Journal of Medicine and Philosophy* 16 (6): 587–92.

Kac, Eduardo. [2000]. (No title). Available at www.ekac.org/gfpbunny.html. Accessed June 22, 2006.

Karpowicz, Phillip. 2003. In defense of stem cell chimeras: a response to "Crossing Species Boundaries." *American Journal of Bioethics* 3 (3): 17–19.

Karpowicz, Phillip, Cynthia B. Cohen, and Derek van der Kooy. 2005. Developing human-nonhuman chimeras in human stem cell research: ethical issues and boundaries. *Kennedy Institute of Ethics Journal* 15 (2): 107–34.

Kass, Leon R. 1971. The new biology: what price relieving man's estate? *Science* 174:779–88.

———. 1985. *Toward a More Natural Science: Biology and Human Affairs.* New York: The Free Press.

———. 1997. The wisdom of repugnance. *New Republic* 216 (22, June 2): 17–26.

———. 2002. *Life, Liberty and the Defense of Dignity: The Challenge for Bioethics.* San Francisco: Encounter Books.

Kingdon, John W. 1984. *Agendas, Alternatives, and Public Policies.* Boston: Little, Brown.

Kobayashi, Nao R. 2003. A scientist crossing a boundary: a step into the bio-ethical issues surrounding stem cell research. *American Journal of Bioethics* 3 (3): 15–16.

Koontz, Dean. 1987. *Watchers.* New York: Berkley Books.

Kopinsky, Nicole E. 2004. Human-nonhuman chimeras: a regulatory proposal on the blurring of species lines. *Boston College Law Review* 45:619–66.

Kurzweil, Ray. 2005. *The Singularity Is Near: When Humans Transcend Biology.* New York: Viking.

Lamb, Gregory M. 2005. A mix of mice and men. *Christian Science Monitor,* March 23. Available at www.cbsnews.com/stories/2005/03/23/tech/print-able682509.shtml. Accessed March 2, 2007; site now discontinued.

Lanza, R.P., J.B. Cibelli, and M.D. West. 1999. Human therapeutic cloning. *Nature Medicine* 5:975–77.

Lavieri, Robert R. 2007. The ethical mouse: be not like Icarus. *American Journal of Bioethics* 7 (5): 57–58.

Ledford, Heidi. 2009. Hybrid embryos fail to live up to stem-cell hopes. *Nature* 457:642–43.

Legislation Review Committee. 2005. Legislation review of Australia's Prohibition of Human Cloning Act 2002 and Research Involving Human Embryos Act 2002. Available at www.lockhartreview.com.au/reports.html. Accessed March 1, 2007; site now discontinued.

Levin, Yuval. 2003. The paradox of conservative bioethics. *The New Atlantis* 1 (spring): 53–65.

Lewis, C. S. 1996. *The Abolition of Man.* New York: Simon & Schuster.

Liger. n.d. Available at http://en.wikipedia.org/wiki/Liger. Accessed August 18, 2006.

Liger.org. 2009. Why Are Ligers Bigger than Tigons? Available at www.Liger.org. Accessed June 30, 2009.

Lomax, Geoffrey, and Susan Stayn. 2008. Similarities and differences among stem cell research policies: opportunities for policymakers, patients, and researchers. *Medical Research Law & Policy Report* 7 (21): 695–98.

Macklin, Ruth. 2003. Dignity is a useless concept. *British Medical Journal* 327:1419–20.

———. 2006. The new conservatives in bioethics: who are they and what do they seek? *Hastings Center Report* 36 (1): 34–43.

Manning, Francis C. R. 2000. Biotechnology: A scientific perspective. In *The International Politics of Biotechnolgy*, edited by Alan Russell and John Vogler, 13–29. Manchester: Manchester University Press.

Markarjan, D. S., E. P. Isakov, and G. I. Kondakov. 1974. Intergeneric hybrids of the lower (42-chromosome) monkey species of the sukhumi monkey colony. *Journal of Human Evolution* 3 (3): 247–55.

Mauron, Alex, and Jean-Marie Thevoz. 1991. Germ-line engineering: a few European voices. *Journal of Medicine and Philosophy* 16 (6): 649–66.

Mayr, Ernst. 1982. *The Growth of Biological Thought: Diversity, Evolution, and Inheritance.* Cambridge, MA: Harvard University Press.

McDermott, Rose. 2004. The feeling of rationality: the meaning of neuroscientific advances for political science. *Perspectives on Politics* 2 (40): 691–706.

McKibben, Bill. 2003. *Enough: Staying Human in an Engineered Age.* New York: Henry Holt and Company.

McLaren, Anne. 2007. Free-range eggs? *Science* 316:339.

Melo-Martin, Inmaculada de. 2008. Chimeras and human dignity. *Kennedy Institute of Ethics Journal* 18 (4): 331–46.

Melton, Douglas A., George Q. Daley, and Charles G. Jennings. 2004. Altered nuclear transfer in stem-cell research—a flawed proposal. *New England Journal of Medicine* 351 (27): 2791–92.

Midgley, David, ed. 2005. *The Essential Mary Midgley.* New York: Routledge.

Midgley, Mary. 2000. Biotechnology and monstrosity: why we should pay attention to the "yuk factor." *Hastings Center Report* 30 (5): 7–15.

———. 2004. *The Myths We Live By.* New York: Routledge.

Mirkes, Renee. 2006. Is it ethical to generate human-animal chimeras? *National Catholic Bioethics Quarterly* 6 (1): 109–30.

Modell, Stephen M. 2007. Approaching religious guidelines for chimera policy-making. *Zygon* 42 (3): 629–41.

Moreno, Jonathan. 2006. President Bush's "hybrid" problem. February 16. Available at http://www.americanprogress.org. Accessed June 18, 2008.

Muotri, Alysson R., Kinichi Nakashima, Nicholas Toni, et al. 2005. Development of functional human embryonic stem cell-derived neurons in mouse brain. *Proceedings of the National Academy of Sciences* 102 (51): 18644–48.

National Centre for the Replacement, Refinement and Reduction of Animals in Research. n.d. About NC3Rs. Available at www.nc3rs.org.uk. Accessed December 26, 2006.

National Council of Churches USA. n.d. "Fearfully and Wonderfully Made: A Policy on Biotechnologies." Available at www.ncccusa.org/pdfs/BioTechPolicy .pdf. Accessed on March 9, 2008.

National Institutes of Health. 1994. *Final Report of the Human Embryo Research Panel.* September 27. Bethesda, MD: National Institutes of Health.

———. 2009. "National Institutes of Health Guidelines on Human Stem Cell Research." July 6, 2009. Available at http://stemcells.nih.gov/policy/2009/ guidelines.htm. Accessed on July 7, 2009.

National Institutes of Health, Recombinant DNA Advisory Committee. 1985. Points to consider in the design and submission of human somatic-cell gene therapy protocols. August 19. *Federal Register* 50 (160): 33463–64.

National Institutes of Health. Office of the Director. 2001. "Notice of Criteria for Federal Funding of Research on Existing Human Embryonic Stem Cells and Establishment of NIH Human Embryonic Stem Cell Registry." November 7. Available at www.grants.nih.gov/grants/guide/notice_files/NOT-OD-02-013. html. Accessed on December 4, 2001.

National Research Council of the National Academies. 2002. *Animal Bio-technology: Science-Based Concerns.* Washington, DC: National Academies Press.

National Research Council and Institute of Medicine. 2007. 2007 Amendments to the National Academies' Guidelines for Human Embryonic Stem Cell Research. Washington, DC: The National Academies Press.

———. 2008. 2008 Amendments to the National Academies' Guidelines for Human Embryonic Stem Cell Research. Available at www.nap.edu/catalog/12260.html. Accessed August 20, 2008.

Nelson, James Lindemann. 2008. Respecting boundaries, disparaging values. *American Journal of Bioethics* 8 (12): 33–34.

NIH cash boosts bid for more knockout mice. 2006. *Nature* 441:921.

Nuffield Council on Bioethics. 2005. *The Ethics of Research Involving Animals*. London: Nuffield Council on Bioethics. Available at www.nuffieldbioethics. org. Accessed June 22, 2006.

Nussbaum, Martha C. 2004. Beyond "compassion and humanity." In *Animal Rights: Current Debates and New Directions*, edited by Cass R. Sunstein and Martha C. Nussbaum, 299–320. New York: Oxford University Press.

———. 2008. Human dignity and political entitlements. In *President's Council on Bioethics, Human Dignity and Bioethics: Essays Commissioned by the President's Council on Bioethics*. 351–80. Washington, DC. March 2008.

Okie, Susan. 2005. Stem-cell research—signposts and roadblocks. *New England Journal of Medicine* 353:1–8.

O'Rourke, P. Pearl, Melinda Abelman, and Kate Gallin Herrernan. 2007. Establishing institutional oversight for human embryonic stem cell research: creating an ESCRO committee. *Medical Research Law & Policy Report* 6 (15): 416–23.

Panthera Hybrid. Available at http://en.wikipedia.org/wiki/Panthera_hybrid. Accessed August 18, 2006.

Parliament of the Commonwealth of Australia. 2006a. Prohibition of Human Cloning for Reproduction and the Regulation of Human Embryo Research Amendment Bill 2006. Bill No. 06160. October 19. Available at http://parlinfo .aph.gov.au/parlInfo/download/legislation/bills/s533_act/toc_pdf/0616080 .pdf;fileType=application%2Fpdf. Accessed December 5, 2006.

———. 2006b. Prohibition of Human Cloning for Reproduction and the Regulation of Human Embryo Research Amendment Bill 2006. Bill No. 06160. October 19. Explanatory Memorandum. Available at http://parlinfo.aph.gov .au/parlInfo/download/legislation/ems/s533_ems_7a7c9382-2edd-45a8-a630-5ac37b4d3fe6/upload_pdf/06160rem.pdf;fileType=application%2Fpdf. Accessed December 5, 2006.

Pennisi, Elizabeth. 2006. Mining the molecules that made our mind. *Science* 313:1908–11.

Peters, Ted. 2006. The return of the chimera. *Theology and Science* 4 (3): 247–59.

Piccinini, Patricia. 2003. We Are Family, Venice Biennale-Roslyn Oxley9 Gallery. Available at www.roslynoxley9.com.au/artists/31/Patricia_Piccinini/249. Accessed September 20, 2006.

Pinker, Steven. 2008. The Stupidity of Dignity. *New Republic* 238 (9, May 28): 28–31.

Pollack, Andrew. 2006. Firm reports stem cell use for making of insulin. *New York Times*, October 20, A18.

President's Council on Bioethics. 2003a. *Beyond Therapy: Biotechnology and the Pursuit of Happiness.* New York: Regan Books.

———. 2003b. Transcript of Meeting, Washington DC. Session 2: Toward A "Richer Bioethics": Chimeras and the Boundaries of the Human. October 16. Available at http://bioethicsprint.bioethics.gov/transcripts/oct03/session2 .html. Accessed July 7, 2005.

———. 2004. *Reproduction and Responsibility: The Regulation of New Bio-technologies.* Washington, DC: President's Council on Bioethics.

———. 2005a. *Alternative Sources of Human Pluripotent Stem Cells.* White Paper. Available at www.bioethics.gov. Accessed January 5, 2006.

———. 2005b. Transcript of Meeting, Washington, DC. Session 5: Human Dignity as a Bioethical Concept. December 9. Available at http://bioethicsprint.bioethics .gov/transcripts/dec05/session5.html. Accessed March 16, 2007.

———. 2005c. Transcript of Meeting, Washington, DC. Session 6: Human-Animal Chimeras. March 4. Available at http://bioethicsprint.bioethics.gov/ transcripts/march05/session6.html. Accessed July 5, 2005.

Qui, Jane. 2006. Mighty mouse. *Nature* 444:814–16.

Rachels, James. 2004. Drawing lines. In *Animal Rights: Current Debates and New Directions,* edited by Cass R. Sunstein and Martha C. Nussbaum, 162–74. New York: Oxford University Press.

Random Samples. 2002. NDArt. *Science* 296:43.

Reston, James Jr. 2006. *Fragile Innocence: A Father's Memoir of His Daughter's Courageous Journey.* New York: Harmony Books.

Ridley, Mark. 1996. *Evolution.* 2nd ed. Cambridge, MA: Blackwell Science, Inc.

Rifkin, Jeremy. 1998. T*he Biotech Century: Harnessing the Gene and Remaking the World.* New York: Penguin Putnam Inc.

Robbins, Jim. 2007. Out west, with the buffalo, roam some strands of undesirable DNA. *New York Times,* January 9, D3.

Robert, Jason Scott. 2006. The science and ethics of making part-human animals in stem cell biology. *FASEB Journal* 20:838–45.

Robert, Jason Scott, and Francoise Baylis. 2003. Crossing species boundaries. *American Journal of Bioethics* 3 (3): 1–13.

———. 2005. Stem cell politics: the NAS prohibitions pack more bark than bite. *Hastings Center Report* 35 (6): 15–16.

Robertson, John A. 1994. *Children of Choice: Freedom and the New Reproductive Technologies.* Princeton, NJ: Princeton University Press.

———. 2006. Compensation and egg donation for research. *Fertility and Sterility* 86 (6): 1573–75.

Rogers, Lesley J., and Gisela Kaplan. 2004. All animals are *not* equal: the interface between scientific knowledge and legislation for animal rights. In *Animal Rights: Current Debates and New Directions,* edited by Cass R. Sunstein and Martha C. Nussbaum, 175–202. New York: Oxford University Press.

Rollin, Bernard E. 2003. Ethics and species integrity. *American Journal of Bioethics* 3 (3): 15–17.

———. 2007a. Of mice and men. *American Journal of Bioethics* 7 (5): 55–57.

———. 2007b. On chimeras. *Zygon* 42 (3): 643–47.

Roussant, Janet. 2004. Embryonic stem cells in perspective. In *Handbook of Stem Cells. Volume 1,* edited by Robert Lanza, John Gearhart, Brigid Hogan, et al., xxi–xxiii. Burlington, MA: Elsevier Academic Press, 2004.

Russell, William, and Rex Burch. 1992. *The Principles of Humane Experimental Technique.* New York: Hyperion Books.

Sagoff, Mark. 2003. Transgenic chimeras. *American Journal of Bioethics* 3 (3): 30–31.

Savulescu, Julian, 2003. Human-animal transgenesis and chimeras might be an expression of our humanity. *American Journal of Bioethics* 3 (3): 22–25.

Savulescu, Julian, and Loane Skene. 2008. The kingdom of genes: why genes from animals and plants will make better humans. *American Journal of Bioethics* 8 (12): 35–38.

Schaub, Diana J. 2006. Chimeras: from poetry to science. *National Catholic Bioethics Quarterly* 6 (1): 29–35.

Schulman, Adam. 2008. Bioethics and the question of human dignity. In *President's Council on Bioethics, Human Dignity and Bioethics: Essays Commissioned by the President's Council on Bioethics,* 3–18. Washington, DC.

Scott, Christopher Thomas. 2006. *Stem Cell Now: From the Experiment That Shook the World to the New Politics of Life.* New York: Pi Press.

Shreeve, Jamie. 2005. The other stem-cell debate. 42. *New York Times Magazine,* April 10.

Siegel, Andrew W. 2003. The moral insignificance of crossing species boundaries. *American Journal of Bioethics* 3 (3): 33–34.

Silver, Lee M. 1997. *Remaking Eden.* New York: Avon Books.

———. 2006. *Challenging Nature: The Clash of Science and Spirituality at the New Frontiers of Life.* New York: HarperCollins Publishers.

Singer, Peter. 1990. *Animal Liberation.* 2nd ed. New York: A New York Review Book.

———. 2004. Ethics beyond species and beyond instincts: a response to Richard Posner. In *Animal Rights: Current Debates and New Directions,* edited by Cass

R. Sunstein and Martha C. Nussbaum, 78–92. New York: Oxford University Press.

Singleton, Rivers. 2000. Transgenic Animals: An Overview. In *Encyclopedia of Ethical, Legal and Policy Issues in Biotechnology,* edited by Thomas J. Murray and Maxwell J. Mehlman, 1088–98. New York: John Wiley & Sons.

Spar, Debora. 2007. The egg trade—making sense of the market for human oocytes. *New England Journal of Medicine* 356 (13): 1289–91.

Species. n.d. Available at http://en.wikipedia.org/wiki/Species. 1–10. Accessed July 25, 2006.

State of the union: the president's speech. 2006. *New York Times,* February 1, A1.

Stock, Gregory. 2002. *Redesigning Humans: Our Inevitable Genetic Future.* Boston: Houghton Mifflin.

Streiffer, Robert. 2005. At the edge of humanity: human stem cells, chimeras, and moral status. *Kennedy Institute of Ethics Journal* 15 (4): 347–70.

———. 2006. Emerging issues in human embryonic stem cell research: chimeras. In The National Academies, Institute of Medicine. *Human Embryonic Stem Cell Research Advisory Committee Public Symposium: Emerging Issues in Human Embryonic Stem Cell Research.* November 7–8. Washington, DC. Available at http://dels.nas.edu/bls/stemcells/symposium2006.shtml. Accessed November 7, 2006.

———. 2008. Informed consent and federal funding for stem cell research. *Hastings Center Report* 38 (3): 40–47.

Sunstein, Cass R., and Martha C. Nussbaum, eds. 2004. *Animal Rights: Current Debates and New Directions.* New York: Oxford University Press.

Svendsen, Clive. 2006. Emerging issues in human embryonic stem cell research. In The National Academies, Institute of Medicine. *Human Embryonic Stem Cell Research Advisory Committee Public Symposium: Emerging Issues in Human Embryonic Stem Cell Research.* November 7–8. Available at http://dels.nas.edu/bls/stemcells/symposium2006.shtml. Accessed November 17, 2006.

Takahashi, K., K. Tanabe, M. Ohnuki, et al. 2007. Induction of pluripotent stem cells from adult human fibroblasts by defined factors. *Cell* 131 (5): 861–72.

Tester, Jason. 2006. Human-animal hybrid T-shirt. Available at http://boingboing.net/2006/02/01/humananimal_hybrid_t.html. Accessed April 4, 2007.

Tigon. n.d. Available at http://en.wikipedia.org/wiki/Tigon. Accessed August 18, 2006.

Transgenic drug gets the go-ahead in Europe. 2006. *Nature* 441:681.

Transhumanism. n.d. Available at http://en.wikipedia.org/wiki/Transhumanism. Accessed October 20, 2006.

Travis, John. 1992. Scoring a technical knockout in mice. *Science* 256:392–94.

Turney, Jon. 1998. *Frankenstein's Footsteps: Science, Genetics and Popular Culture.* New Haven, CT: Yale University Press.

U.K. Department of Health. 2000a. A report from the Chief Medical Officer's Expert Group reviewing the potential of developments in stem cell research and cell nuclear replacement to benefit human health. In *Stem Cell Research: Medical Progress with Responsibility.* London: Department of Health.

———. 2000b. Government response to the recommendations made in the Chief Medical Officer's Expert Group Report "Stem Cell Research: Medical Progress with Responsibility."

———. 2006. Review of the Human Fertilisation and Embryology Act: Proposals for Revised Legislation (including establishment of the Regulatory Authority for Tissue and Embryos). Available at www.dh.gov.uk/en/publicationsand-statistics/publications/publicationspolicyandguidance/dh_073098. Accessed January 24, 2007.

———. 2007a. Correspondence from Ted Webb, Deputy Director Scientific Development and Bioethics, to Kate Lawrence, Clerk to the Joint Committee on the Draft Human Tissue and Embryos Bill, 12 June. Available at www.parliament.uk/documents/upload/070621DoH.pdf. Accessed May 30, 2009.

———. 2007b. Hybrids and chimeras: a report on the findings of the Consultation. October. Available at www.hfea.gov.uk/docs/Hybrids_Report.pdf. Accessed June 28, 2008.

U.K. House of Commons. Science and Technology Committee. 2005. *Human Reproductive Technologies and the Law. Fifth Report of Session 2004–05* (Volume 1). Available at http://www.publications.parliament.uk/pa/cm200405/cmselect/cmsctech/7/702.htm. Accessed March 6, 2006.

———. 2007. *Fifth Report of Session 2006–07, Government Proposals for the Regulation of Hybrid and Chimera Embryos, HC 272-1.* London: The Stationery Office Limited. Available at www.publications.parliament.uk/pa/cm200607/cmselect/cmsctech/272/272i.pdf. Accessed March 3, 2009.

U.K. Human Fertilisation and Embryology Act 2008. 2008. Available at www.uk-legislation.hmso.gov.uk/acts/acts2008a. Accessed December 12, 2008.

United Kingdom. Parliament. Select Committee on Animals in Scientific Procedures. 2002. Chapter 8: Genetically Modified Animals. Available at www.publications.parliament.uk/pa/ld200102/ldselect/ldanimal/150/15001.htm. Accessed November 3, 2006.

United Kingdom. Parliament. Select Committee on Science and Technology. 2007a. Memorandum 6. Submission from The Wellcome Trust/Cancer

Research UK Gurdon Institute of Cancer and Developmental Biology, University of Cambridge.

———. 2007b. Memorandum 7. Submission from Biosciences Federation.

———. 2007c. Memorandum 9. Submission from Scottish Council on Human Bioethics.

———. 2007d. Memorandum 12. Submission from Institute of Biology.

———. 2007e. Memorandum 14. Submission from North-East England Stem Cell Institute (NESCI).

———. 2007f. Memorandum 15. Submission from Dr. Robin Lovell-Badge.

———. 2007g. Memorandum 20. Submission from Dr. Lyle Armstrong, University of Newcastle upon Tyne.

———. 2007h. Memorandum 21. Submission from Christian Action Research and Education.

———. 2007i. Memorandum 23. Submission from Christian Medical Fellowship.

University of Wisconsin Stem Cell and Regenerative Medicine Center. 2008. Stem Cell Research Oversight (SCRO) Committee. Available at www.stemcells.wisc.edu/escro.html. Accessed December 23, 2008.

U.S. Senate. 2005a. Human Chimera Prohibition Act of 2005. S. 659. 109th Congress. 1st Session. March 17.

———. 2005j. Human Chimera Prohibition Act of 2005. S. 1373. 109th Congress. 1st Session. July 11.

Urie, Kimbery A., Alison Stanley, and Jerold D. Friedman. 2003. The humane imperative: a moral opportunity. *American Journal of Bioethics* 3 (3): 20.

van der Meer, Miriam. 2002. Transgenesis and animal welfare: implications of transgenic procedures for the well-being of the laboratory mice. Dissertation Abstract. Proefschrift Universiteit Utrecht. Available at http://igitur-archive.library.uu.nl/dissertations/2002-0409-121120/UUindex.html. Accessed November 3, 2006.

Vestal, Christine. 2007. Embryonic stem cell research divides states. Available at www.stateline.org/live/details/story?contentID=218416. Accessed June 21, 2007.

Vogel, Gretchen. 2006. Team claims success with cow-mouse nuclear transfer. *Science* 313:155–56.

———. 2008. U.K. approves new embryo law. *Science* 322:663.

Wade, Nicholas. 2005. Chimeras on the horizon, but don't expect centaurs. *New York Times*, May 3, D1.

———. 2006. New DNA test is yielding clues to Neanderthals. *New York Times*, November 16, A1.

Walters, LeRoy. 1987. Ethics and new reproductive technologies: an international review of committee statements. *Hastings Center Report* 17:3S–9S.

Walters, LeRoy, and Julie Gage Palmer. 1997. *The Ethics of Human Gene Therapy.* New York: Oxford University Press.

Warnock, Mary. 1985. *A Question of Life: The Warnock Report on Human Fertilisation and Embryology.* Oxford: Basil Blackwell.

Washington University in St. Louis. 2005. Policies and procedures. Human embryonic stem cell research guidelines. Revised November 29. Available at www.wustl.edu/policies/humanembryonicstemcellresearchguidelines.html. Accessed June 27, 2007.

Wells, H. G. 1993. *The Island of Doctor Moreau: A Variorum Text,* edited by Robert M. Philmus. Athens, GA: University of Georgia Press.

When two fuse with one. 2007. *Nature* 446:473.

White House. Office of the Press Secretary. 2009. Executive Order 13435. Removing Barriers to Responsible Scientific Research Involving Human Stem Cells. March 9. Available at http://www.whitehouse.gov/the_press_office/ Removing-Barriers-to-Responsible-Scientific-Research-Involving-Human-Stem-Cells. Accessed on March 17, 2009.

Wilford, John Noble. 2006. Neanderthals in gene pool, study suggests. *New York Times,* November 9, A21.

Wise, Steven M. 2002. *Drawing the Line: Science and the Case for Animal Rights.* Cambridge, MA: Perseus Books.

———. 2004. Animal rights, one step at a time. In *Animal Rights: Current Debates and New Directions,* edited by Cass R. Sunstein and Martha C. Nussbaum, 19–50. New York: Oxford University Press.

Witherly, Jeffre L., Galen P. Perry, and Darryl L. Leja. 2001. *An A to Z of DNA Science: What Scientists Mean When They Talk about Genes and Genomes.* Cold Spring Harbor, NY: Cold Spring Harbor Laboratory Press.

Wood, Cynthia. n.d. The not-so-legendary chimera. Available at www.damn-interesting.com/?p=412. Accessed September 18, 2006.

Working Group on Interspecific Chimeric Brains. 2005. Phoebe R. Berman Bioethics Institute, Johns Hopkins University. Available at http://www.hopkins-medicine.org/bioethics/scope/projects/workinggroupinterspecificch.html. Accessed June 21, 2005.

Yu, J., M. A. Vodyanik, K. Smuga-Otto, et al. 2007. Induced pluripotent stem cell lines derived from human somatic cells. *Science* 318 (5858): 1917–20.

Index